RETHINKING RISK ASSESSMENT

Rethinking Risk Assessment

The MacArthur Study of Mental Disorder and Violence

by
JOHN MONAHAN
HENRY J. STEADMAN
ERIC SILVER
PAUL S. APPELBAUM
PAMELA CLARK ROBBINS
EDWARD P. MULVEY
LOREN H. ROTH
THOMAS GRISSO
STEVEN BANKS

OXFORD
UNIVERSITY PRESS
2001

OXFORD
UNIVERSITY PRESS

Oxford   New York
Athens   Auckland   Bangkok   Bogotá   Buenos Aires   Calcutta
Cape Town   Chennai   Dar es Salaam   Delhi   Florence   Hong Kong   Istanbul
Karachi   Kuala Lumpur   Madrid   Melbourne   Mexico City   Mumbai   Nairobi
Paris   São Paulo   Shanghai   Singapore   Taipei   Tokyo   Toronto   Warsaw

and associated companies in
Berlin   Ibadan

Copyright © 2001 by Oxford University Press, Inc.

Published by Oxford University Press, Inc.
198 Madison Avenue, New York, New York 10016
http://www.oup-usa.org

Library of Congress Cataloging-in-Publication Data
Rethinking risk assessment : the MacArthur study of mental disorder and violence /
by John Monahan . . . [et al.].
p. ; cm.   Includes bibliographical references and index.
ISBN 0-19-513882-1
1. MacArthur Violence Risk Assessment Study.   2. Dangerously mentally ill—United States.
3. Violence—United States.   4. Risk assessment—United States.   5. Insane—Commitment and
Detention—United States.
I. Monahan, John, 1946–   II.
MacArthur Violence Risk Assessment Study.
[DNLM: 1. Mental Disorders—diagnosis.   2. Violence—psychology.
3. Mental Disorders—psychology.   4. Risk Assessment—methods.   5. Risk Factors.
WM 141 R438 2000]   RC569.5.V55 R47 2000   616.89'075—dc21   00-062434

9 8 7 6 5 4 3 2 1

Printed in the United States of America
on acid-free paper

PREFACE

Despite enormous advances in the diagnosis and treatment of mental disorder in recent decades, the social stigma associated with having a mental disorder remains great. Why is this so? According to the Surgeon General's first Report on Mental Health (1999), "The answer appears to be fear of violence: people with mental illness, especially those with psychosis, are perceived to be more violent than in the past" (p. 7). This perception has become a driving force—often *the* driving force—in mental health law and policy in the United States and throughout the world.

This book addresses the violence that people with mental disorder sometimes engage in. More specifically, it addresses how that violence can be anticipated, the first step toward prevention. Our goal is to offer mental health professionals a clinical tool that can improve both the accuracy and the efficiency of the violence risk assessments that they are increasingly called on to make. We believe that judges, lawyers, and legal scholars also will find our substantive conclusions of interest and that researchers will find our methods to be innovative and to be useful in other contexts as well.

We review in this book a great deal of recent research on a wide array of variables claimed to be risk factors for violence. We focus most heavily, however, on one study, the MacArthur Violence Risk Assessment Study. This book brings together and integrates all of the recently published results of that project and includes findings presented for the first time.

The Violence Risk Assessment Study was the largest of three major empirical thrusts of the MacArthur Research Network on Mental Health and the Law. A second emphasis concerned the competence of people with mental disorder to make decisions regarding their mental health treatment (e.g., Grisso & Appelbaum, 1998) or the adjudication of criminal charges against them (e.g., Otto, Poythress, Nicholson, Edens, Monahan, Bonnie, Hoge, & Eisenberg, 1998). A final concern dealt with the role played by coercion in the administration of mental health services (e.g., Lidz, Hoge, Gardner, Bennett, Monahan, Mulvey, & Roth, 1995). In addition, the Network supported more circumscribed work on violence risk communication (e.g., Slovic, Monahan, & MacGregor, 2000) and on work disability and the law (Bonnie & Monahan, 1997). A complete list of the Network's research can be found on its website, http://macarthur.virginia.edu/

The Violence Risk Assessment Study was supported by the John D. and Catherine T. MacArthur Foundation and by National Institute of Mental Health grant R01 49696. The Study was nurtured at every step by the remarkably capable and supportive staff of the MacArthur Foundation: Laurie Garduque, Robert Rose, Idy Gitelson, and Ruth Runeborg. Denis Prager and William Bevan played key roles in the study's early stages.

We are deeply indebted to the other members of the Research Network on Mental Health and the Law, including Shirley S. Abrahamson, Richard J. Bonnie, Pamela S. Hyde, Stephen J. Morse, Paul Slovic, and David B. Wexler, for their insights on every phase of the research. We thank Seth Leon, Nan Brady, and, especially, Roumen Vesselinov, for their significant contributions in data management and analysis. A draft of this book was carefully reviewed by Renée Binder, Joel Dvoskin, Stephen Hart, and Kirk Heilbrun. The book is better for their insights.

We also gratefully acknowledge the contributions of William O'Connor, Ph.D., and Deirdre Klassen, Ph.D., as the site directors in Kansas City, as well as the site coordinators, research clinicians, and field interviewers at each of the three data collection sites: Kimberly Ackerson, Ph.D., Tamara Anderson, Bruce Dembling, Ph.D., Carolyn Hill-Fotouhi, M.A. Jan Meymaris, Dawn O'Day, and Kim Trettel Smith, M.A., in Worcester; Jennifer King, Ray Milke, Debra Murray, Lorrie Rabin, Ph.D., Chelsea Ruttenburg, Carol Schubert, M.P.H., and Esther VonWaldow, M.S.W. in Pittsburgh; and Julie Applegate, Ph.D., Ron Dancy, Heather Fitz-Charles, Lisa Johnson-Sharpe, Ph.D., Lisa Kuhn, Susan Kuntz, Walter Janzen, M.A.,

Brian Lindhardt, M.A., Becca Matthews, Lisa Rogers, Melba Small, Aileen Utley, Ph.D., and Rick Wright in Kansas City.

Much more may be learned from the rich information on mental disorder and violence that we have assembled in the MacArthur Violence Risk Assessment Study. The complete data set has been archived and is available to researchers free of charge. See the Network's website for information on how to access it.

Charlottesville, Va.   J. M.

CONTENTS

RETHINKING RISK ASSESSMENT

1

VIOLENCE RISK ASSESSMENT: THE LAW AND THE SCIENCE

Beliefs about the causes of mental disorder have changed over the centuries, but the belief that mental disorder predisposes many of those suffering from it to behave violently has endured. Indeed, this belief appears to have increased in intensity in the past several decades, despite many educational campaigns designed to allay public apprehension (Phelan, Link, Stueve, & Pescosolido, 2000). The more a member of the general public believes that mental disorder and violence are associated, the less he or she wants to have an individual with a mental disorder as a neighbor, friend, colleague, or family member (Link, Phelan, Bresnahan, Stueve, & Pescosolido, 1999b).

These perceptions are reflected both in formal policies toward people with mental disorders and in the public's expectations about the role of mental health professionals in ensuring the safety of the community. Violence risk assessment now is widely assumed by policy makers and the public to be a core skill of the mental health professions and plays a pivotal role in mental health law throughout the world.

Before the late 1960s, commitment to psychiatric facilities was justified primarily by a paternalistic concern for people who were seen to be "in need of treatment." Beginning in the late 1960s, however, public protection began to dominate as a rationale for commitment, and risk of behavior harmful to others—called "dangerousness" in statutes and court decisions—became a primary focus of clinical and legal attention (Appelbaum, 1988, 1994). Despite a refocusing of standards in a few jurisdictions to reemphasize the more diffuse "mental or physical deterioration" that disorder can precipitate, risk of physical harm has remained firmly embedded in mental health law as a prime rationale for various forms of involuntary intervention. For example, the American Psychiatric Association's Model State Law on Civil Commitment (1983), based heavily on the work of Stone (1975), follows Roth (1979) in explicitly contemplating the commitment to a mental hospital of several types of people with mental disorder, including those "likely to cause harm to others."

More recently, the American Bar Association's *National Benchbook on Psychiatric and Psychological Evidence and Testimony* (1998) stated that courts rely on information in the form of clinical risk assessments when making decisions regarding institutionalization "because courts are ultimately responsible for making these decisions and though the information may remain open to challenge, it is the best information available. The alternative is to deprive fact finders, judges and jurors of the guidance and understanding that psychiatrists and psychologists can provide" (p. 49).

It is not only as a standard for involuntary hospitalization that risk of violence is a cornerstone issue in mental health law. Involuntary outpatient commitment statutes frequently include "dangerousness" as a commitment standard (Swartz, Swanson, Wagner, Burns, Hiday & Borum, 1999). Less legally formal procedures for "community supervision and monitoring" and for the intensive administration of community-based mental health services are also often predicated on a perceived risk of violence (Dennis & Monahan, 1996). In addition, discharge from forensic hospitals after a finding of not guilty by reason of insanity is almost always contingent on a prediction that violence is unlikely to occur (Steadman, McGreevy, Morrissey, Callahan, Robbins, & Cirincione, 1993; Silver, 1995). Finally, the imposition of tort liability on mental health professionals who negligently fail to anticipate and avert a patient's violence to others has become commonplace in many jurisdictions (Monahan, 1993; Gutheil & Appelbaum, 2000).

CLINICAL RISK ASSESSMENT: OUTCOMES

None of the laws and policies just described is predicated on the assumption that *all* people with mental disorder will be violent. Rather, they are premised on the belief that some people with mental disorder will be violent and others will not, and, furthermore, on the expectation that mental health professionals can distinguish with a reasonable degree of accuracy between "dangerous" and "nondangerous" cases of mental disorder (Monahan, 2000a; Mossman, 2000; Mullen, 1997, 2000); and therein has long lain the rub.

Early research on the accuracy of clinicians at predicting violent behavior to others was reviewed by Monahan (1981). Five studies (Kozol, Boucher, & Garofalo, 1972; Steadman & Cocozza, 1974; Cocozza & Steadman, 1976; Steadman, 1977; Thornberry & Jacoby, 1979) were available as of the late 1970s. The conclusion of that review was that

> psychiatrists and psychologists are accurate in no more than one out of three predictions of violent behavior over a several-year period among institutionalized populations that had both committed violence in the past (and thus had high base rates for it) and who were diagnosed as mentally ill. (p. 47)

Only two studies of the validity of clinicians' predictions of violence in the community have been published since that time (for reviews, see Blumenthal & Lavender, 2000; Monahan, 2000b). Sepejak, Menzies, Webster, & Jensen (1983) studied court-ordered pretrial risk assessments and found that 39% of the defendants rated by clinicians as having a "medium" or "high" likelihood of being violent to others were reported to have committed a violent act during a 2 year follow-up period compared with 26% of the defendants predicted to have a "low" likelihood of violence (p. 181, note 12), a statistically significant difference, but not a large one in absolute terms.

More recently, Lidz, Mulvey, & Gardner (1993) took as their subjects male and female patients being examined in the acute psychiatric emergency room of a large civil hospital. Psychiatrists and nurses were asked to assess potential patient violence to others over the next 6 month period. Patients who elicited professional concern regarding future violence were more likely to be violent after discharge (53%) than were patients who had not elicited such concern (36%). The accuracy of clinicians' predictions of violence by male patients, but not by female patients, significantly exceeded chance levels. (For important studies assessing risk of violence within inpatient mental health facilities, see McNiel & Binder [1994] and McNiel, Sandberg, & Binder [1998]).

CLINICAL RISK ASSESSMENT: PROCESS

Mulvey and Lidz (1985) have argued that to study the *outcome* of clinical prediction before studying the *process* of clinical prediction is to "put the cart before the horse" (p. 213). They stated that

> it is only by knowing "how" the process occurs that we can determine . . . the strategy for improvement in the prediction of dangerousness. Addressing this question requires systematic investigation of the possible facets of the judgement process that could be contributing to the observed low predictive accuracy. (p. 215)

Along these lines, Segal, Watson, Goldfinger, and Averbuck (1988a, b) observed clinicians evaluating over 200 cases at several psychiatric emergency rooms. Observers coded each case on an 88 item index called Three Ratings of Involuntary Admissibility (TRIAD). Global ratings of patient "dangerousness" were completed by each clinician. The TRIAD scores correlated highly with overall clinical ratings of dangerousness.

> Symptoms most strongly related to [clinical judgments of] danger to others in our sample were irritability and impulsivity, but there were also consistent moderate associations with formal thought disorder, thought content disorder, and expansiveness as well as weaker but consistent significant correlations with impaired judgment and behavior and inappropriate affect. (1988b, p. 757)

Similarly, Menzies and Webster (1995) studied the clinical decision making process regarding risk for a large group of Canadian mentally disordered offenders. They concluded that "previous violence, alcohol use, presentation of anger and rage, lack of agreeability, and tension during the interviews were the main contributors to the resulting decisions" (p. 775).

In the research program of Mulvey and Lidz (e.g., Mulvey & Lidz, 1985; Lidz, Mulvey, Apperson, Evanczuk, & Shea, 1992), observers trained in speedwriting recorded interviews between clinicians and patients admitted to a hospital's psychiatric emergency room. Clinicians later completed ratings of current and chronic dangerousness in the community. Although a patient's history of violence was the best predictor of clinician ratings, patient hostility and the presence of serious disorder also correlated highly with clinical ratings of current dangerousness. In addition, explicit judgments of the likelihood of future violence were rarely found in actual practice, with this conclusion instead embedded in other decisions about clinical care.

CHOOSING A RESEARCH STRATEGY

Because of the central importance of violence in mental health law and policy throughout the world, and because the state of the science on which those laws and policies rested was so shaky, the MacArthur Research Network on Mental Health and the Law, when it was planning its research agenda in the late 1980s, had little difficulty in choosing violence risk assessment as a core concern. But how best to proceed? More research demonstrating that the outcome of unstructured clinical assessments left a great deal to be desired seemed to be overkill: That horse was already dead. On the other hand, systematic studies unpacking the process by which clinicians made estimates of violence risk were already in progress (e.g., Mulvey & Lidz, 1985), and there was no need to duplicate them. Ultimately, the Network—like others working independently around the same time (e.g., Harris, Rice, & Quinsey, 1993; Webster, Douglas, Eaves, & Hart, 1995)—decided that the way forward in improving risk assessment for community violence was likely to lie not in directly addressing the process of clinical judgment at all, but rather in developing an evidence-based actuarial tool that would inform that judgment.

ACTUARIAL RISK ASSESSMENT

The general superiority of statistical over clinical risk assessment in the behavioral sciences has been known for almost half a century (Meehl, 1954; Grove, Zald, Lebow, Snitz, & Nelson, 2000; Swets, Dawes, & Monahan, 2000). Despite this, and despite a long and successful history of actuarial risk assessment in bail and parole decision making in criminology (Champion, 1994), there have been only a few attempts to develop actuarial tools for the specific task of assessing risk of violence to others among people with mental disorder (for reviews, see Monahan & Steadman, 1994; Borum, 1996;

Douglas, Cox, & Webster, 1999). For example, Steadman and Cocozza (1974), in an early study of mentally disordered offenders, developed a Legal Dangerousness Scale based on the presence or absence of a juvenile record and a conviction for a violent crime, the number of previous incarcerations, and the severity of the current offense. This scale, along with the patient's age, was significantly associated with subsequent violent behavior. Likewise, Klassen and O'Connor (1988a) found that the combination of a diagnosis of substance abuse, prior arrests for violent crime, and young age were significantly associated with arrests for violent crime among male civil patients discharged into the community.

More recently, the Violence Risk Appraisal Guide (VRAG) (Harris et al., 1993; Quinsey, Harris, Rice, & Cormier, 1998; Rice & Harris, 1995b) was developed from a sample of over 600 men from a maximum-security hospital in Canada. All had been charged with a serious criminal offense. Approximately 50 predictor variables were coded from institutional files. The criterion was any new criminal charge for a violent offense, or return to the institution for a similar act, over a time at risk in the community that averaged approximately 7 years after discharge. A series of regression models identified 12 variables for inclusion in the VRAG, including the Hare Psychopathy Checklist—Revised, elementary school maladjustment, and age at the time of the offense (which had a negative weight). When the scores on this actuarial instrument were dichotomized into "high" and "low," the results were that 55% of the group scoring high committed a new violent offense compared with 19% of the group scoring low.

Finally, and most recently, Douglas and Webster (1999) reviewed ongoing research on a structured clinical guide that can be scored in an actuarial manner to assess violence risk, the "HCR-20," which consists of 20 ratings addressing Historical, Clinical, or Risk management variables (Webster et al., 1995). Douglas and Webster also reported data from a retrospective study with prisoners, finding that scores above the median on the HCR-20 increased the odds of past violence and antisocial behavior by an average of four times. In another study with civilly committed patients, Douglas, Ogloff, Nicholls, and Grant (1999) found that during a follow-up period of approximately 2 years after discharge into the community, patients scoring above the HCR-20 median were 6 to 13 times more likely to be violent than were patients scoring below the median.

THE EVOLUTION OF THE MACARTHUR VIOLENCE RISK ASSESSMENT STUDY

For the reasons just given, we were convinced, as we began to plan the MacArthur Violence Risk Assessment Study, not only of the importance to mental health law and policy of improving the validity of violence risk assessment but also that the path to achieving this goal lay in an actuarial direction (cf. Buchanan, 1999). We had two core goals: to do the best "science" on violence risk assessment possible and to produce a violence risk assessment "tool" that clinicians in today's world of managed mental health services could actually use. From these initial intellectual commitments, our thinking evolved in stages over the decade it took to plan, execute, and analyze the research. These stages are described in detail in the subsequent chapters of this book, and we briefly introduce them here as a roadmap of what is to follow.

IDENTIFYING GAPS IN METHODOLOGY

As we reviewed the existing studies that had attempted to statistically relate given risk factors or combinations of risk factors to violent behavior among people with mental disorder, we came to the conclusion that almost all suffered from one or more methodological problems: They considered a constricted range of risk factors, often a few demographic variables or scores on a psychological test; they employed weak criterion measures of violence, usually relying solely on arrest; they studied a narrow segment of the patient population, typically males with a history of prior violence; and they were conducted at a single site (The studies and their methodological difficulties were reviewed in detail by Monahan & Steadman [1994].) Based on this critical examination of existing work, we initially set out to design a piece of research that could, to the greatest extent possible, overcome the methodological obstacles we had identified. We would study a large and diverse array of risk factors. We would triangulate our outcome measurement of violence, adding patient self-report and the report of a collateral informant to data from official police and hospital records. We would study both men and women, regardless of whether they had a history of violence; and we would conduct our study at several sites rather than at a single site.

SELECTING PROMISING RISK FACTORS

It is one thing to want to study a large and diverse array of risk factors. It is another to choose which specific risk factors to study. Although we lacked any comprehensive theory of violence by people with mental disorder from which we could derive hypothesized risk factors (see Reiss & Roth [1993] on the absence of such a theory), recent studies suggested a number of variables that might be potent risk factors for violence among people with a mental disorder. Among those variables were psychopathy, anger, delusions, hallucinations, diagnosis, gender, violent thoughts, child abuse, prior violence, and contextual variables (Monahan & Steadman, 1994). We chose what we believed to be the best of the existing measures of these variables and, when no instrument to adequately measure a variable was available, we commissioned the development of the necessary measure.

From the beginning, we knew it was naive to think that one or a small number of risk factors could accurately predict violence. Like virtually all existing violence risk assessment researchers, we tried to combine many risk factors using a main effects regression model. The results achieved with this standard statistical technique were not, however, appreciably better than those that others had obtained using far less elaborate (and costly) data-collection procedures. The use of a main effects regression model, on reflection, seemed to imply that the effect of particular risk factors on the occurrence of violence is the same for all people with mental disorder. Such a model did not capture the richness of the relationships we were observing among risk factors as they related to violence. We began to take a different analytic tack.

USING TREE-BASED METHODS

Drawing from new work by Gardner, Lidz, Mulvey, and Shaw (1996a, b), we developed violence risk assessment models based on classification tree rather than linear regression methods. A classification tree approach reflects an interactive and contingent model of violence, one that allows many different combinations of risk factors to classify a person at a given level of risk. The particular questions to be asked in any assessment grounded in this approach depend on the answers given to prior questions. Factors that are relevant to the risk assessment of one person may not be relevant to the risk assessment of another person. This contrasts with a regression approach in which a common set of questions is asked of everyone being assessed, and every answer is weighted to produce a score that can be used for purposes of categorization.

Yet, as others have concluded (e.g., Gottfredson & Gottfredson, 1980), we found that the predictive accuracy achieved by using a classification tree was no better than that provided by a standard main effects regression model. Additional steps were necessary to substantially improve predictive accuracy.

CREATING DIFFERENT CUT-OFFS FOR HIGH AND LOW RISK

The first step was to abandon the expectation that we could classify all people into a high or a low violence risk group. Rather than relying on the standard single threshold for distinguishing among cases, we decided to employ two thresholds—one for identifying high risk cases and one for identifying low risk cases. Recalling Shah (1978), we assumed that inevitably there would be cases that fall between these two thresholds, cases for which any actuarial prediction scheme is incapable of making an adequate assessment of high or low risk. The degree of risk presented by these intermediate cases cannot be statistically distinguished from the base rate of the sample as a whole (hence, we refer to these cases as constituting an "average risk" group). By focusing actuarial attention on cases at the more extreme ends of the risk continuum, we thought that we might increase predictive accuracy for the cases we designated as extreme (Menzies, Webster, & Sepejak, 1985; McNiel 1998).

REPEATING THE CLASSIFICATION TREE

The second step we took to increase the predictive accuracy of a classification tree was to reanalyze those cases designated as "average risk." That is, all people not classified into groups designated as either high or low risk in the standard classification tree model were pooled together and reanalyzed. The logic here was that the people who were not classified in the first iteration of the analysis might be different in some significant ways from the people who were classified and that the full set of risk factors should be available to generate a new classification tree specifically for the people who were not already classified as high or low risk. The process of pooling and reanalyzing cases was continued until no additional groups of subjects could be classified as high or low risk. We referred to the resulting classification tree model as an "iterative" classification tree (ICT).

When we analyzed our data using two cut-offs rather than one, and using an iterative rather than a standard classification tree, the improvement in predictive accuracy we were able to achieve was substantial.

COMBINING MULTIPLE RISK ESTIMATES

Finally, we were concerned that the success of the ICT at assessing violence risk might be due, in part, to overfitting the data (i.e., to capitalization on chance). This concern led us to estimate several different ICT models in an attempt to obtain multiple risk assessments for each case. That is, we chose a number of different risk factors to be the lead variable on which a classification tree was constructed. In attempting to combine these multiple risk estimates, we began to conceive of each separate risk estimate as an indicator of the underlying construct of interest, violence risk. The basic idea was that patients who scored in the high risk category on many classification trees were more likely to be violent than were patients who scored in the high risk category on fewer classification trees. (Analogously, patients who scored in the low risk category on many classification trees were less likely to be violent than were patients who scored in the low risk category on fewer classification trees.) The use of multiple risk estimates from different ICTs — it is impossible to resist the temptation to use the word "forest" here — resulted in a further and equally substantial boost in predictive accuracy. Multiple models of risk were much more accurate than was any single model of risk.

CONCLUSIONS

The use of violence risk assessment has become pervasive in mental health law around the world, yet research continues to indicate that clinicians' unaided abilities to perform this task are modest at best. The MacArthur Violence Risk Assessment Study is grounded in the resurgence of interest in actuarial approaches to assessing violence risk. We identified gaps in existing research methodology and selected promising risk factors. We decided to use tree-based rather than main-effects analytic methods. We chose separate cut-off scores for identifying high risk and low risk cases, and we repeated the tree to classify as many cases as possible into these extreme risk categories. Finally, we generated a number of different classification trees to see how consistently patients performed and whether the consistency of this performance related to violence risk. Cumulatively, these steps produced the results that we originally had hoped for.

The methodology of the MacArthur Violence Risk Assessment Study is described in detail in Appendix A. The subsequent chapters of this book characterize the violence we observed (Chapter 2), summarize our findings on key risk factors — both "criminological" (Chapter 3) and "clinical" (Chapter 4) — and explain the development of iterative classification trees (Chapter 5) and the ways that these trees can be combined (Chapter 6). We conclude (Chapter 7) with a discussion of the implications of our work for the practice of risk assessment and risk management.

2

VIOLENCE AMONG PATIENTS IN THE COMMUNITY

A clinician assessing the likelihood of future violence must inevitably start with the simple, but far from straightforward, question of exactly what constitutes "patient violence." As pointed out repeatedly about a variety of clinical prediction tasks (Meehl, 1954; Garb, 1998), it is difficult to reach a high level of predictive accuracy without a clear picture of what is being predicted, whether that prediction is done using actuarial or clinical methods.

This initial task of defining the violence of concern, however, rests substantially on whether the clinician has an accurate perspective about patient violence in general. It is necessary to know how the violence potential of the patient being assessed compares with the base rates of different types of violence in the group of patients being seen as well as how the rates of these behaviors may be expected to change over time after discharge from the hospital. This kind of information forms the frame of any judgment about what types of violence might be anticipated or avoided (Skeem & Mulvey, in press b).

Unfortunately, information about the nature of patient violence is rather limited, mainly because researchers have used a variety of generally weak measures of violence in the community. Many researchers have simply used arrest or recommitment to the hospital as proxies for violence, and those studies that have used self-reports of patients have often asked broad questions that do not allow for in-depth descriptions of separate incidents (e.g., Swanson, Holzer, Ganju, & Jono, 1990). A few studies have used more involved patient reports and the reports of others who are familiar with the activities of the patient (e.g., Lidz, Mulvey, & Gardner, 1993; Link, Andrews, & Cullen, 1992; Swanson, Borum, Swartz, & Hiday, 1999). Only rarely have researchers provided a contextualized view of patient violence in an effort to examine the dynamics underlying these events (e.g., Estroff & Zimmer, 1994; Toch & Adams, 1994). Moreover, these different types of measurement have been used with a variety of patients, ranging from hospitalized inpatients, to discharged civil patients, to select groups of forensic patients or those on outpatient commitment orders. The result is a blurred picture of patient violence.

There are some notable consistencies and inconsistencies across these studies. There is evidence that patient violence occurs more frequently with family members or close acquaintances in either the patient's or someone else's home and that most incidences of patient violence reported involve actions no more serious than fistfights, if that (Newhill, Mulvey, & Lidz, 1994; Steadman et al. 1998; Swanson, Borum, Swartz, & Hiday, 1999). There is still considerable controversy, however, about whether mental illness produces a distinct form of serious violence in mentally disordered people (Taylor, 1993; Steury & Choinski, 1995).

The MacArthur Violence Risk Assessment study moves the field forward by providing a more detailed view of patient violence than has generally been available in past research. This view gives the clinician a backdrop against which to consider the potential violence of a patient. In addition, it provides researchers with a starting point for future investigations that consider patient violence in a more differentiated and potentially informative fashion.

SOURCES OF INFORMATION

The methods employed in the MacArthur Violence Risk Assessment Study are described in full in Appendix A. In brief, admissions were sampled from acute civil inpatient facilities in Pittsburgh, PA, Kansas City, MO, and Worcester, MA. We selected English-speaking patients between the ages of 18 and 40 years who were of white, African-American, or Hispanic ethnicity and who had a chart diagnosis of thought or affective disorder, substance abuse, or personality disorder.

The patient was interviewed in the hospital by both a research interviewer and a research clinician. A wide variety of risk factors were assessed, including dispositional factors (e.g., age and gender), historical factors (e.g., mental hospitalization and violence history), contextual factors (e.g., social supports and stress), and clinical factors (e.g., diagnosis and specific symptoms). All 134 risk factors that were assessed are listed in Appendix B.

Three sources of information were used to ascertain the occurrence and details of a violent incident in the community. Interviews with patients, interviews with collateral individuals (i.e., persons named by the patient as someone who would know what was going on in his or her life), and official sources of information (arrest and hospital records) were all coded and compared. The patients and collaterals were interviewed five times (every 10 weeks) over 1 year from the date of hospital discharge.

TYPES OF VIOLENCE

For the analyses reported here, the types of violent incidents are often collapsed into two broad categories. The first is labeled "violence" to indicate its more serious nature; it includes acts of battery that resulted in physical injury; sexual assaults; assaultive acts that involved the use of a weapon; or threats made with a weapon. For an incident to be coded as "weapon threat," the subject had to have a weapon in hand at the time of the incident; telling someone that a weapon would be obtained or having one available but not in hand (e.g., in a drawer of the room) did not constitute a weapon threat.

The second category is called "other aggressive acts," a group that includes incidents of battery that did not result in injury. Verbal threats are not included as other aggressive acts. Previous studies (mostly those of inpatient violence) have often included verbal threats as violent incidents, but our judgment was that these behaviors were both difficult to document reliably in the community and of limited usefulness. We decided to examine acts in which a patient was placing another in danger or had decided to take some physical action against another person. As a result, care should be used when comparing the rates reported here with those found by other investigators.

The categorization system using these two groups (violence and other aggressive acts) draws a line at the infliction of injury or the threat of considerable, credible harm. We have made this distinction to provide a more differentiated view of patient violence and to avoid misrepresenting the scope of this issue in the lives of mentally ill individuals. Using a definition that "clumps" all incidents under a highly inclusive rubric of patient violence, one might conclude that violence among mental patients is almost commonplace. A highly restrictive definition, on the other hand, might underestimate the importance of this problem. A view of these incidents in at least two categories lets the reader see the range of these behaviors and allows for a more balanced assessment of the role of violence in patients' lives. Moreover, the patterns and relationships between certain case characteristics and the occurrence of "patient violence" may be very different depending on where the boundaries of the outcome measure are drawn. The factors related to more serious violence may or may not be the same ones associated with less serious violence.

UNITS OF ANALYSIS

The sources we chose provide a rich picture of the violent incidents in the lives of these patients in the community. Details are available about such things as the seriousness of the violence, who was involved, and where the incident occurred. Because repeated interviewing was done and the follow-up period covered 1 year after hospital discharge, there is also information about the patterns of violent behavior over time. For our purposes here, we examined this information in three ways, and each method of describing the data has a different advantage for informing policy and future research.

First, the data can be viewed with the incident as the unit of analysis. Collapsing across all incidents, we can identify phenomena such as how many of these incidents occurred among family members and how many involved the use of weapons. This approach provides information about the range and types of incidents in which patients were involved, without a concern for the involvement of any individual patient in multiple incidents. It provides a broad view of the landscape of patient violence in a sample of approximately 1000 patients in the year after hospital discharge.

A second approach is to consider the individual patient as the unit of analysis and to classify or characterize each patient according to his or her involvement with violence. For example, patients could be classified as having engaged in some form of violence or not during a particular follow-up period or as being repetitively violent or not. This way of examining the data separates patients into groups based on a summary variable related to their violent behavior, and it allows for the identification of individual case characteristics related to these groupings. This approach is the one most commonly taken in prior research in this area, because it has the potential for providing information about how to sort patients according to their likelihood to engage in violence during a given time period after clinical assessment (Mulvey, Blumstein, Cohen, 1986).

Finally, the data can be examined for patterns over time. Subjects vary in their frequency and timing of involvement with violence. Consideration of factors such as the time to the first violent event or how incidents distribute over the follow-up period provides leads about when patients may be at greater or lesser risk for violence after discharge. These individual patterns may also reveal different subgroups of patients with distinctive risk characteristics.

DESCRIPTION OF VIOLENT INCIDENTS

Table 2.1 describes the types of violent incidents reported over the entire 1 year follow-up period. As shown, the highest proportion of all incidents of violence across the 1 year follow-up period (49%) involved the patient hitting or beating up someone. There was, however, a considerably high level of weapon use and threat (29%). Most incidents involving just other aggressive acts (74%) were ones with slapping, grabbing, shoving, or throwing objects.

Most of the violence and other aggressive acts observed involved close relationships in home environments. It is clear that spouses, boyfriends/girlfriends, and other family members are most likely to be those who are in-

TABLE 2.1. Types, Targets, and Locations of Violence and Other Aggressive Acts Over the 1 Year Follow-Up Period

	Violence (%)	Other Aggressive Acts (%)
A. Types of Violence and Other Aggressive Acts		
	(n = 608)	(n = 2668)
Throwing object	12.0	74.0
Push-grab-shove		
slap		
Kick-bite-choke	49.3	22.0
Hit-beat up		
Force sex	5.3	0.0
Weapon threat	29.3	0.0
Weapon use		
Other, type unknown	4.1	3.9
B. Targets of Violence and Other Aggressive Acts		
	(n = 558)	(n = 2366)
Family	51.1	61.9
Spouse	23.3	23.3
Girlfriend/Boyfriend	13.8	15.2
Parental figure	2.5	3.6
Child	2.5	6.7
Other family	9.0	13.1
Friend/Acquaintance	35.1	27.2
Stranger	13.8	10.9
C. Locations of Violence and Other Aggressive Acts		
	(n = 552)	(n = 2362)
Subject's home	43.3	60.8
Other residence	25.7	13.9
Street/Outdoors	21.6	14.9
Bar	4.5	4.4
Outpatient clinic	0.7	1.1
Workplace	0.5	1.7
Other	3.7	3.2

volved in incidents with patients. In addition, most violent incidents (69%) and other aggressive acts (75%) occurred in the patient's or another person's residence.

There were few incidents that occurred in public settings, other than on the street. The limited number of incidents of workplace violence or other aggressive acts at a workplace could be related to the relatively low level of employment found in this sample (only about 55% reported part-time or full-time employment during any one follow-up period), but it might also indicate a situational influence of this type of setting. Sorting out this effect would require having and examining data regarding the actual amount of time spent in work settings. The proportion of incidents that occurred on the street may reflect the process of individuals being asked to leave public settings as encounters escalated. Incident accounts were also reviewed and coded for the types of factors that appeared to precipitate the conflict, the presence or absence of particular situational features, and the outcomes of the incident (see Steadman & Silver, 2000). We were interested in knowing such things as how the participants came together, how many of these incidents involved the use of alcohol, and whether the patient reported taking his or her medication at the time. Consideration of these factors gives a richer snapshot of the situational context of the reported incidents than is usually available.

Most of the violent incidents seemed to occur in the normal flow of a patient's daily life. In the 473 violent incidents for which information is available, most (56%) occurred during some regularly scheduled event (e.g., a meal, a recreational activity), whereas others resulted from a chance encounter with the co-participant (24%). In only 13% of these incidents did the subject or co-participant seek out the other person with the intent of harming them.

Table 2.2 summarizes several situational features associated with the incidents recorded. Information about each of these features was not available for all of the incidents, and the percentage figure indicates the proportion of incidents having this feature where information was available.

As found in other studies of violence in the general population (White, 1997), alcohol use appears to be a regular feature of these incidents. In addition, although these data do not allow for an assessment of the specific effect of medication compliance on the likelihood of violence (see Chapter

TABLE 2.2. Behaviors of the Patient at the Time of the Violent Incident

Patient Activity	Total No.	%
Drinking just before the incident	499	54.1
Using illegal drugs just before the incident	488	23.0
Prescribed a psychotropic medication at the time of the incident*	494	49.4
Having delusional thoughts at the time of the incident	434	7.4
Hearing voices at the time of the incident	466	5.2
Taken to a psychiatric hospital as a result of the incident	476	6.7
Arrested as a result of the incident	479	15.7

* This is the number of incidents in which the patient reported that a medication had been prescribed for that time period. It is unknown how many people may have been prescribed medications but did not report this fact.

7), it is striking that about a one-fourth of the violent incidents (54% of the 49% where the patient reports having a medication prescribed) involve a situation in which the patient was not taking a prescribed medication. Very few of the incidents (less than 10%), however, occurred when the patient was displaying active psychotic symptoms (i.e., delusions or hallucinations) (cf. Taylor, 1998), and only a small proportion resulted in the patient being arrested.

The interviewers also asked how the fight ended. In almost half (45%) of the incidents for which this information is available (n = 463), it was reported that the subject or co-participant simply left the scene or the people involved just stopped fighting when "enough" injury had been inflicted. In another sizable proportion (37%), the incident stopped because either a third party (in 19%) or the police (in 18%) intervened. Apparently, only a small proportion of these incidents are ever recorded in an official record anywhere.

INCIDENTS LINKED TO PATIENTS

There are several ways to identify each patient with a particular type of incident. Perhaps the most elemental, and informative, method is simply to

TABLE 2.3. Proportion of Patients with Follow-Up Violence or Other Aggressive Acts by Information Source (n = 951)

Information Source	% with Violence by Information Source	Cumulative %* with Violence	% with Other Aggressive Acts by Information Source	Cumulative % with Other Aggressive Acts
Agency records	4.5	4.5	8.8	8.8
Subject	22.4	23.7	44.6	47.7
Collateral	12.7	27.5	31.8	56.1

*Cumulative = agency records alone (row 1), agency records plus patient self-report (row 2), and agency records plus patient self-report plus collateral report (row 3).

see if the patient committed a violent or other aggressive act during a particular 10 week period or during the entire follow-up period. When we initially examined the data for this outcome, we were struck by how much the source of information shaped the prevalence rate of cases with violent incidents.

Table 2.3 shows the percentage of cases that would be classified as having a violent incident during the entire follow-up period, depending on the data source used to make this determination. Based on these results, it makes quite a difference whether one relies on self-reports or official records when estimating the prevalence of violent incidents in this sample. Clearly, use of all of the available sources provides a much more complete and detailed picture of the number and types of incidents (and this approach is used in the rest of the analyses reported here). Using official records only, we would have estimated that only 4.5% of our sample had a violent incident during the follow-up period. Using official records, patient reports, and collateral reports together raises this estimate to 27.5%, indicating that violent incidents occurred in a substantial proportion of the patients studied.

It is also clear that most of the reported incidents came from patient self-reports. If we had relied solely on patient self-report, we would have identified 22.4% of the patients as having a violent incident, and the use of collateral reports added only an additional 3.8% of cases identified. Thus, although the use of collateral reports did increase the "yield" of violent cases by approximately 17%, this approach required considerable effort and cost to achieve this return. It is important to note, however, that this research

design provided a near ideal situation to minimize underreporting of violence (e.g., no repercussions from staff). Other designs may produce more
inclinations to underreport, making the collateral data more valuable.

There are a substantial number of subjects in the sample who had more than
a single act of violence or other aggressive act. Tables 2.4 and 2.5 show the number of subjects who had repeated incidents of violence or other aggressive acts.
Almost half (45%) of those with violent incidents (n = 262) had more than one
such incident. Of those with other aggressive acts (n = 529), two-thirds (67%)
had more than one of these incidents during the 1 year period.

Given the repetitive nature of much of the reported violence and other
aggressive acts, it is useful to characterize cases according to the most serious
incident and first act reported for each subject. As shown in Table 2.6,
subjects can contribute only one incident to the overall distribution of incidents. These summaries provide information that can be particularly informative when related to that provided in Table 2.1, in which all incidents
are summarized. Comparing the incident characteristics in Table 2.6 with
those in Table 2.1 (where subjects can each contribute numerous incidents
to the distribution) tells us how much that allowing these repeated observations into the picture might cloud our view of what patient violence generally looks like. Removal of these repeated incidents would change our view
of the contours of patient violence if the repetitively violent patients consis-

TABLE 2.4. Numbers of Violent Acts Committed by Discharged Patients
During 1 Year Follow-Up Period

Number of Violent Incidents	Number of Discharged Patients
0	689
1	145
2	50
3	29
4	17
5	8
6	4
7 or more	9
Total incidents = 608	Total persons = 262

TABLE 2.5. Numbers of Other Aggressive Acts Committed by Discharged
Patients During 1 Year Follow-Up Period

Number of Other Aggressive Acts	Number of Discharged Patients
0	422
1	174
2	102
3	57
4	43
5	31
6	19
7	18
8	11
9	14
10–19	35
20–75	25
Total incidents = 2,668	Total persons = 529

tently engaged in particular forms of violence. If individuals who did repeat
violence, for example, were disproportionately likely to have incidents that
occurred at home, then limiting these subjects to just one incident would
reduce the proportion of incidents that occurred in residences from that seen
in the previous analysis of all incidents.

Table 2.6 suggests that limiting each case to just one incident (whether
the most serious one or the first one) does not change the general profile of
the types of act, targets, and locations of incidents. Most incidents still involve fights or weapon threats and occur with family members in residences.
There is a slight increase in the proportion of incidents that involve friends/
acquaintances from that reported in Table 2.1, indicating that repetitively
violent patients may be more likely to have repeated domestic violence, but
this difference is far from dramatic. Overall, these results suggest that the
repetitively violent patients and those committing one or few acts are involved generally in the same types of incidents. In short, repetitively violent
patients appear to be just performing more of the same types of violent acts
done by those patients who engage in only one violent act.

TABLE 2.6. Types, Targets, and Locations of Violence Over the 1 Year Follow-Up Period

	Most Serious Violent Act (%)	First Violent Act (%)
A. Types of Violence and Other Aggressive Acts		
	(n = 262)	(n = 262)
Throwing object	11.8	15.3
Push-grab-shove		
Slap		
Kick-bite-choke	45.4	51.5
Hit-beat up		
Force sex	4.6	2.7
Weapon threat	34.0	24.8
Weapon use		
Other, type unknown	4.2	5.7
B. Targets of Violence and Other Aggressive Acts		
	(n = 251)	(n = 249)
Family	43.0	44.6
Spouse	17.9	19.3
Girlfriend/Boyfriend	7.2	8.4
Parental figure	3.6	3.6
Child	2.8	2.8
Other family	11.6	10.4
Friend/Acquaintance	41.4	40.2
Stranger	15.5	15.3
C. Locations of Violence and Other Aggressive Acts		
	(n = 250)	(n = 249)
Subject's home	45.6	45.3
Other residence	18.8	18.6
Street/Outdoors	26.4	27.5
Bar	4.4	4.5
Outpatient clinic	0.8	0.8
Workplace	0.4	0.4
Other	3.6	2.8

It is also instructive to see how involvement in violence or other aggressive acts changes over the 1 year follow-up period. Tables 2.7, 2.8, and 2.9 summarize how many patients engaged in violence or other aggressive acts at each follow-up period and the average number of incidents reported for each patient at each of these points. It is clear from Table 2.7 that fewer of the subjects in the sample are involved in violence and other aggressive acts as the year after discharge progresses, with the number of patients with reported incidents dropping off noticeably 20 weeks after discharge. It also appears that there is a drop in the rate of incidents per patient over the follow-up periods. Table 2.8 shows that there are fewer cases with multiple violent or other aggressive acts during each successive follow-up period. Table 2.9 goes on to show that, among those with violent or aggressive acts during each follow-up period, the rate of these acts also drops over time. Taken together, these results indicate that the patients in this sample are most likely to be involved in violence during the first 20 weeks after discharge and that the likelihood of repeated incidents of violence or other aggressive acts also decreases after this initial postdischarge period.

The decreases in the overall prevalence and rate of involvement in violence over the follow-up periods could result from several different processes. The most obvious explanation might be that patients simply become less likely to engage in violence the longer they are in the community. This explanation, however, rests on the assumption that the decrease reflects actual patient behavior over time and is not a methodological artifact.

Three artifactual explanations could produce this result. First, there is the possibility of greater attrition by violent patients. In other words, we could have lost more violent patients for follow-up interviews over the course of the study and thus achieved lower violence rates overall with each follow-up period. Second, violent patients might have been off the streets more as the study progressed. People who committed violent acts might have been in a jail or hospital and therefore unable to continue their violence in the later follow up periods. Finally, reporting bias might have occurred with repeated interviewing. Subjects might have realized that reporting violence lengthened the interview and, to avoid this, might have censored their reports of violence.

TABLE 2.7. Prevalence of Cases with Violence and Other Aggressive Acts

			Total Patient Sample	
	n	*Violence (%)*	*Other Aggressive Acts Only (%)*	*Violence or Other Aggressive Acts (%)*
Pre-hospital*	1136	17.4	25.8	43.2
Follow-up No. 1	852	13.5	25.2	38.7
Follow-up No. 2	818	10.3	22.7	33.0
Follow-up No. 3	755	6.9	18.8	25.7
Follow-up No. 4	739	7.6	18.0	25.6
Follow-up No. 5	726	6.3	14.2	20.5
One-year aggregate	951	27.5	33.0	60.6

* Self-report only.

TABLE 2.8. Prevalence of Cases with Multiple Violent and Other Aggressive Acts During Each Follow-Up Period

		Total Patient Sample	
	n	*Two or More Violent Acts (%)*	*Two or More Other Aggressive Acts Only (%)*
Follow-up No. 1	852	4.2	15.5
Follow-up No. 2	818	2.7	14.3
Follow-up No. 3	755	2.0	9.4
Follow-up No. 4	739	1.6	8.5
Follow-up No. 5	726	1.2	6.2
One-year aggregate	951	12.3	37.3

TABLE 2.9. Number of Violent and Other Aggressive Acts per Subject

| | Total Patient Sample | | | | | | | | |
| | Violent Acts | | | Other Aggressive Acts Only | | | Violent or Other Aggressive Acts | | |
	Number of Subjects	Number of Acts	Mean per Subject	Number of Subjects	Number of Acts	Mean per Subject	Number of Subjects	Number of Acts	Mean per Subject
Follow-up No. 1	115	202	1.8	283	894	3.2	330	1096	3.3
Follow-up No. 2	84	153	1.8	238	734	3.1	270	887	3.3
Follow-up No. 3	52	113	2.2	170	388	2.3	194	501	2.6
Follow-up No. 4	56	83	1.5	159	372	2.3	189	455	2.4
Follow-up No. 5	46	57	1.2	125	280	2.2	149	337	2.3
One year	262	608	2.3	529	2668	5.0	576	3276	5.7

We tested each of these possible artifactual explanations and found that none of them accounted for the observed drop in overall prevalence over the 1 year follow-up period (the exact tests are reported in Steadman et al., 1998). We looked at those patients who participated in all five follow-up interviews and saw the same type of drop-off in prevalence (see Table 2.10). We also modeled the effects of time out of the community and attrition and found that correcting for these processes changed the prevalence estimates only slightly. Finally, we examined other parts of the interview that should have shown comparable reductions in reporting if the subjects were selectively reporting information to shorten the interview and found no such patterns.

As we state in Steadman et al. (1998, p. 400), "substantive hypotheses to account for this decline are legion." Positive influences from treatment or social support may become influential over time in the community after hospitalization. Alternatively, periods of active symptomatology related to violence may be unaffected by treatment, still persist well past the hospitalization period, and simply subside over the 1 year follow-up period.

TABLE 2.10. Prevalence of Violent and Other Aggressive Acts for Subjects with No Missing Violence Data

	Patient Sample with no Missing Violence Data (n = 536)		
	Violent Acts (%)	Other Aggressive Acts Only (%)	Violent or Other Aggressive Acts (%)
Pre-hospital*	14.4	24.3	38.6
Follow-up No. 1	11.2	23.7	34.9
Follow-up No. 2	7.1	23.5	30.6
Follow-up No. 3	6.0	17.5	23.5
Follow-up No. 4	6.7	17.0	23.7
Follow-up No. 5	5.8	14.2	20.0
One-year aggregate	25.2	34.7	59.9

* Self-report only.

INDIVIDUAL PATTERNS OF VIOLENCE OVER TIME

We also examined the timing of violent incidents. Although much attention is paid in the research literature to the *prevalence* of violence among patients during a given time period, little is known about the *imminence* of violent behavior, that is, the extent to which violence occurs early in time following hospital discharge. In addition, although a great deal of effort has been spent trying to identify risk factors that help to sort cases according to prevalence, little is known about the extent to which there exist different subgroups of patients who exhibit different violence trajectories over time. Yet, it seems plausible that a patient who commits a violent act immediately after hospital discharge is at higher "risk" of violence than a patient who does not commit a violent act until the 20th week (or 20th month) after discharge. Furthermore, it would be of great practical value to clinicians to be able to identify subgroups of patients who are likely to exhibit specific patterns of violence over time.

The mean number of days to a first violent act among subjects who engaged in violence during the 1 year follow-up period was 130; the median was 106. The difference in the mean and median values indicates that the distribution of time to first incident is skewed to the left, with most subjects having their initial incident relatively soon in the year after discharge. This regularity is illustrated in Figure 2.1, which shows the hazard rate of the time to the first violent incident, measured as the number of days from hospital discharge. The curve indicates the likelihood that a patient will have an initial violent incident within a given time period after discharge. Clearly, patients are at higher risk for their initial incident within the first 150 days after discharge.

We also looked for empirically identifiable subgroups with different patterns of violence over the follow-up period. It was our suspicion that there might be a group of patients who had a flurry of incidents in the period right after discharge and another group of "late bloomers" who had violent incidents at some time further into the follow-up period. We looked for these different patterns of violence over time, or "trajectories," using a semiparametric model developed by Nagin and his colleagues (Nagin & Land, 1993; Land & Nagin, 1996; Nagin & Tremblay, 1999). In this approach, the data are examined for the presence of empirically discernible groups of subjects

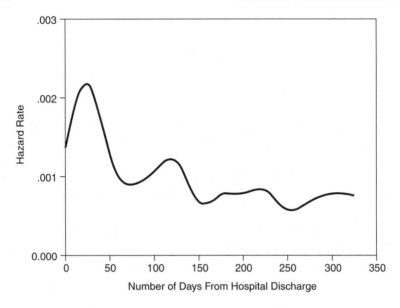

FIGURE 2.1. Hazard rate for time to first violent incident.

with different patterns of violent incidents over the follow-up period. The patterns of violence are not stated *a priori*, but instead the data are examined for any possible patterns that might exist. For example, if there were clear groups of patients who dropped off early in their violence and others whose violence accelerated steadily, the model would identify the presence of these "trajectories" of behavior over the follow-up period.

This analysis showed that a model containing only two distinct subgroups best described the data. One group was composed of patients who had no involvement in violent incidents. The other was a group of patients whose involvement in violence decreased over time. In other words, the patients who engaged in violence all followed the same general pattern of less involvement in violence over time. There did not appear to be any distinct subgroups of patients with different patterns of offending over the follow-up period.

CONCLUSIONS

This overview of patient violence in the community provides a rich set of details about the numbers and types of incidents reported as well as patterns of behavior over time. There are notable regularities about the violence in the lives of these patients. There are also a number of questions that still need to be addressed in future work.

Perhaps the most notable observation is simply that violence is not a rare event in the lives of many patients. About one-fourth of the patients reported a violent incident during the 1 year follow-up period, and about half of the patients who had violent incidents had more than one. Moreover, the patients in this sample were willing to talk about these incidents, but if we had not asked about them, most of these incidents would have gone undocumented. Clinicians asking about violence may find it to be more of a factor in community adjustment than is generally assumed. More systematic and routine documentation and exploration of the details of prior violent incidents should have a payoff for clinicians.

It is important to keep in mind, however, that the level of reported violence in this sample does not necessarily indicate that discharged patients are, simply by virtue of who they are, more dangerous than their community neighbors. In another report from these data, we have shown that patients in this sample who did not have a co-occurring substance abuse disorder were no more likely to have a violent incident than were individuals living in the same neighborhoods (Steadman et al., 1998). The discharged patients were, however, more likely than their neighbors to be involved in substance abuse.

In addition, we have seen that neighborhood conditions exert a clear influence on the likelihood of engaging in violence among these patients over and above the individual characteristics of the patient (see Chapter 3). The violence reported here among these patients, like other violence, occurs in a social context, and consideration of the role of this context is necessary to understand the meaning of the overall prevalence figures reported here.

In future examinations of the dynamics of patient violence, it will probably be useful to consider another simple observation from the data reported here. That is, the violence reported by these patients has many of the same characteristics of violence reported in nonmentally ill samples. Family members and close acquaintances are most likely to be involved in the violent incidents, most incidents occur in someone's home, and alcohol seems to play a large role. In addition, most of the reported violent events involving patients occur in the course of regular, daily activities. The scenario of the violent patient setting out on a mission to harm someone else is not the common one. Instead, the incidents occur in the stream of events of everyday life. Thus, in general, it seems that patient violence may be most reasonably conceptualized as violence involving people with mental illness rather than a distinct form of irrational behavior.

Finally, these findings highlight the need to provide adequate services to patients in the time period shortly after hospital discharge if the goal is to reduce the likelihood of violence. Patients were at highest risk for involvement in violence in the first 20 weeks after hospital discharge, and this pattern seemed to hold rather uniformly across the whole sample (i.e., there were no subgroups of patients who followed an identifiable, different pattern). The implication of these findings for service provision is clear. More focused care in the community in the months immediately after discharge seems a worthwhile investment for reducing violence (see Chapter 7).

In the rest of the analyses reported in this book, we have chosen to examine violence in terms of whether the patient was involved in a violent incident (as defined in this chapter) during the first 20 weeks out of the hospital or during the entire follow-up period. As shown in this chapter, this is only one possible characterization of what it means to be involved in violence. We could have looked at rates of violence over time or involvement in particular types of violent acts, such as those against family members. Future research using more differentiated depictions of violence like these would certainly be valuable. It is possible that given variables are predictive for particular forms of violence, but not for others. Such possibilities warrant investigation.

Our choice of outcomes for the rest of the analyses here, however, is based on simplicity and relevance. Everyone can understand what it means if a patient is involved in an incident of a certain seriousness within a given time period. In the rest of the book, we examine those factors that appear to be related to patient violence during the year after hospital discharge because this makes maximal use of our data set. We look at the 20 week period immediately after discharge because this represents the time period during which both patients appear to be at highest risk for violence and clinicians or a mental health system might reasonably take steps to reduce the likelihood of violence after discharge.

3

TESTING "CRIMINOLOGICAL" RISK FACTORS

To date, guidance for clinicians as to how to assess violence risk among people with mental disorders has largely taken the form of highlighting a number of "key" risk factors to which clinicians should attend. Monahan (1981), for example, identified 10 risk factors for violence that were claimed to have clinical relevance. More recently, Webster et al. (1995) have compiled a list of 20 risk factors that they believe contribute to a comprehensive clinical risk assessment.

The MacArthur Violence Risk Assessment Study provided an opportunity to test the relationship between a large number of putatively pivotal risk factors and subsequent violence. Patients were assessed on a wide range of variables culled from both available theories of and research on violence and mental disorder and the accumulated experience of clinicians (Steadman et al., 1994). This culling process identified 134 potential risk factors (see Krae-mer, Kazdin, Offord, Kessler, Jensen, & Kupfer [1997] for terminology in this area) that were measured in the study. The predictive association between each of these variables, taken singly, and violence during the first 20 weeks after hospital discharge is presented in Appendix B. There it can be seen that odds ratios for individual variables ranged from approximately 1.0 (number of prior hospitalizations) to approximately 4.0 (psychopathy).[1]

---

[1] An odds ratio indicates the number of times the odds is increased for every unit change in the risk factor. For example, if the odds ratio for the effect of male gender on violence is

Before presenting in subsequent chapters our principal findings about how these individual variables can be combined to form a valid tool for violence risk assessment, we describe in this and the following chapter what we have learned regarding a number of these individual variables. We selected the variables to highlight based on their clinical and theoretical prominence in the field of violence risk assessment. We chose to elaborate both on variables that have long been considered in the criminological literature to be prime risk factors for violence and on variables whose status as important risk factors for violence has been advanced by clinicians (see Wessely & Taylor, 1991). The "criminological" variables we address in this chapter are gender, prior violence and criminality, childhood experiences, and neighborhood. The "clinical" variables we consider in the following chapter are diagnosis, psychopathy, delusions, hallucinations, violent thoughts, and anger (see also Bonta, Law, & Hanson, 1998).

We emphasize that the goal in this chapter and in the next is not to isolate an individual variable or small group of variables that by themselves are a sufficient indicator of high violence risk among all groups of patients. Such a goal, we argue in Chapters 5 and 6, is unattainable. Rather, we believe that the variables described here are of particular clinical or scholarly interest in their own right, independent of whether they will be combined with many other variables in an actuarial risk assessment instrument.

The basic methodology of the MacArthur Study is presented in Appendix A. We present here only those additional facets of methodology necessary to understand the variable under consideration. Many of the variables addressed here have been the subject of journal articles that one or another of the authors has recently written. In those circumstances, the reader is referred to the published article for methodological details and precise statistical tests. When we use the word "significant" in this chapter and in the next, we mean statistically significant at at least the 0.05 level.

In general, we focus here both on violence during the first 20 weeks after

---

2.0, then the odds of violence for males is twice as great as the odds of violence for females. The "standardized odds ratio" that is also presented in Appendix B expresses the same information except that the change in the odds of violence is for a 1 standard deviation unit change in the risk factor. For example, if the standardized odds ratio for age is 2.0, then the odds of violence increases by a factor of 2 for every standard deviation increase in age.

hospital discharge — that is, the commission of at least one violent act during either of the first two 10 week follow-up periods — and on violence during the full 1 year follow-up period. We selected the first 20 weeks after discharge because that is the period during which rates of violence were at their peak (Chapter 2).

GENDER

That women commit violent acts at a much lower rate than men is a staple in criminology. Women make up 51% of the U.S. population but only 11% of the people arrested for violent crime (Reiss & Roth, 1993). The United States appears to be approximately in the middle of the international distribution of gender ratios in arrest rates for violence, which vary from 5 to 1 to 50 to 1 (Wilson & Herrnstein, 1985). Although gender differences are sometimes less for self-report than for official report (Steffensmeier & Allen, 1996), national crime survey findings closely parallel the arrest record data: 14% of violent offenders were reported by their victims to be women or girls (Greenfeld & Snell, 1999). As Sampson and Lauritsen (1994) concluded, "sex is one of the strongest demographic correlates of violent offending" (p. 19).

It is against the background of this fundamental tenet of criminology that the results of several recent studies of violence by men and women with mental disorder are so striking. Lidz et al. (1993), in a study of persons discharged from short-term psychiatric facilities, found no significant differences in the rates of community violence by male and female patients. Similar results have been reported for violence within mental hospitals (Estroff & Zimmer, 1994). Indeed, the underestimation of the likelihood of violence by women patients has been suggested as a major factor underlying the lack of validity that plagues clinical violence risk assessment (Lidz et al., 1993; McNiel & Binder, 1995). The hypothesis that mental disorder has more of an effect on the violence-potential of women than of men has also received support in the epidemiological literature (Hodgins, 1992; Swanson, Holzer, Ganju, & Jono, 1990; Brennan, Mednick, & Hodgins, 2000). Even where gender differences in violence are not eliminated, the magnitude of those differences appears strongly attenuated when the samples consist of men and women with mental disorder compared to when they consist of men and women without it.

Measures of Violence and Other Aggressive Acts in the MacArthur Study

As discussed in Chapter 2, the criterion measure we used in the MacArthur Violence Risk Assessment Study was divided into two categories of seriousness: *violence* (battery that resulted in physical injury; sexual assaults; assaultive acts that involved the use of a weapon; or threats made with a weapon in hand) and *other aggressive acts* (battery that did not result in physical injury). Although elsewhere in this chapter we generally limit our focus to violence rather than extend it to other aggressive acts, when considering gender we believe that it is important to present findings for both violence and other aggressive acts, as significant and consistent differences between men and women are found along this dimension.

Were There Gender Differences in Violence?

The final sample given a hospital interview consisted of 667 men and 469 women. Although there were no significant gender differences in age, race, or length of hospital stay, there were significant gender differences in diagnosis. Women were more likely than men to have a primary research diagnosis of depression and less likely to have a primary research diagnosis of alcohol/drug abuse or dependence. In addition, among patients without a *primary* research diagnosis of alcohol/drug abuse or dependence, women were significantly less likely than men to have a *co-occurring* research diagnosis of alcohol or drug abuse/dependence (34% of the women and 52% of the men). Women were also less likely to have a *history* of alcohol or drug abuse recorded in the hospital chart (64% for women and 79% for men).

What Was the Relation of Gender to Violence and Other Aggressive Acts?

The proportion of patients with at least one act of violence during the first 20 weeks after discharge from the hospital was 21.4% for the men and 15.2%

for the women, a statistically significant difference. Men were not, however significantly more likely than women to have been violent over the course of the entire 1 year follow-up, period (29.7% for men vs. 24.6% for women). In contrast, the proportion of patients with at least one other aggressive act *only*—that is, another aggressive act *not* accompanied by an act of violence—during the first 20 weeks was 35.2% for the women compared with 27.1% for the men, a statistically significant difference. Women were also significantly more likely to have other aggressive acts during the 1 year follow-up period (30.1% for men vs. 37.0% for women). (To avoid double counting, patients with both violence and other aggressive acts are counted as "violent" in the computation of these rates.)

As shown in Table 3.1, panel A, for both men and women the acts that were coded as violence over the course of the 1 year follow-up period were primarily "kick/bite/choke/hit/beat up" and "weapon threat/weapon use," and the acts that were coded as other aggressive acts were primarily "throwing objects/push/grab/shove/slap." "Throwing objects/push/grab/shove/slap" constituted a significantly higher proportion of women's than of men's violence and a significantly higher proportion of women's than of men's other aggressive acts. "Kick/bite/choke/hit/beat up" constituted a significantly higher portion of men's violence and a significantly higher proportion of men's other aggressive acts.

The targets of both violence and other aggressive acts committed by men and by women were most often family members, followed by friends and acquaintances (Table 3.1, panel B). For both violence and other aggressive acts, the targets of women were significantly more likely to be family members, and the targets of men were significantly more likely to be friends and acquaintances or to be strangers.

The locations of both violence and other aggressive acts committed by men and by women were most often in the subject's home, in the home of another, or outdoors/on the street (Table 3.1, panel C). Women were significantly more likely to have their violence and other aggressive acts take place at home, and men were significantly more likely to have their violence and other aggressive acts take place outdoors/on the street.

To eliminate any bias that may have been introduced in these analyses due to the fact that some of the patients committed multiple acts of violence or other aggressive acts, we reanalyzed the data looking only at the most

TABLE 3.1. Types, Targets, and Locations of Violent and Other Aggressive Acts in 1 Year by Gender

	Violent Acts		Other Aggressive Acts Only	
	Women	Men	Women	Men
A. Types of Violent and Other Aggressive Acts				
	(n = 215)	(n = 393)	(n = 1329)	(n = 1339)
Throw object, push, grab, shove, or slap	15.8	9.9*	79.9	68.2***
Kick, bite, choke, hit, beat up	43.7	52.4*	18.5	25.5***
Forced sex	7.0	4.3	0.0	0.0
Weapon use or threat with weapon in hand	31.2	28.2	0.0	0.0
Other, type unknown	2.3	5.1	1.6	6.3***
B. Targets of Violent and Other Aggressive Acts				
	(n = 210)	(n = 348)	(n = 1203)	(n = 1163)
Family	69.5	39.9***	74.6	48.8***
Spouse	44.3	10.6***	31.8	14.6***
Girlfriend/Boyfriend	8.1	17.2**	19.2	11.0***
Parental figure	1.4	3.2	3.5	3.6
Child	6.2	0.3***	9.0	4.4***
Other family	9.5	8.6	11.2	15.1**
Friend/Acquaintance	26.2	40.5***	20.9	33.6***
Stranger	4.3	19.5***	4.4	17.6***
C. Locations of Violent and Other Aggressive Acts				
	(n = 208)	(n = 344)	(n = 1199)	(n = 1163)
Subject's home	55.8	35.8***	68.2	53.1***
Other residence	20.7	28.8*	12.8	15.0
Street/Outdoors	14.4	25.9***	9.5	20.5***
Bar	3.8	4.9	4.1	4.7
Outpatient clinic	0.5	0.9	0.8	1.5
Workplace	1.0	0.3	0.8	2.6***
Other	3.8	3.5	3.8	2.5

All data are incident-level. Male versus female: * p < .05 ** p < .01 *** p < .001.

serious act for each individual. The reanalysis generally supported the findings reported above (e.g., there were significant differences between men and women in the choice of target, with men more likely to target strangers and less likely to target spouses and children, and in the location of the violence, with men more likely to have outdoor incidents; see Robbins, Monahan, & Silver [2000] for specific findings).

Descriptive data on the contexts preceding and following the violent incidents also showed significant gender differences. Violent acts by women were less likely to have been preceded by alcohol or drug consumption and more likely to occur while psychiatric medications were being taken. In addition, violent acts by women were less likely to result in arrest and less likely to result in someone being sent for medical treatment.

Conclusions Regarding Gender and Violence

Findings from this research that men are no more likely to be violent than women over the course of the 1 year follow-up period differ dramatically from results generally found in the criminological literature, but not from findings of other studies of men and women with a mental disorder. In addition, those gender differences that are observed during the first 20 weeks after hospital discharge can be partially explained by the higher prevalence of co-occurring substance abuse diagnosis in patients who are men.

Although the overall prevalence rates are similar for women and men, there are some substantial gender differences in the quality or context of the violence committed (see Gelles & Straus, 1988). Men are more likely to have been drinking or using street drugs, and less likely to have been taking prescribed psychotropic medication, before committing violence. Women are more likely to target family members and to be violent in the home. The violence committed by men is more likely to result in serious injury—requiring treatment by a physician—than the violence committed by women, and perhaps for that reason men are more likely than women to be arrested after committing a violent act. In general, these findings underscore the necessity for clinicians not to underestimate the likelihood of violence committed by women. That violence committed by women tends to be less "visible" than violence committed by men—occurring disproportionately more against family members, at home, and without response from the police—may indicate that clinicians should be particularly careful to inquire about violence among patients who are women.

PRIOR VIOLENCE AND CRIMINALITY

The field of criminology has repeatedly demonstrated that prior violence and criminality are strongly associated with future violence and criminality (Blumstein, Cohen, Roth, & Visher, 1986). Similar relationships have been found specifically for persons with mental illnesses. For example, presence of a juvenile record has been found to be predictive of adult violence among male psychiatric patients (Steadman & Cocozza, 1974; Klassen & O'Conner, 1988a). Likewise, prior adult offending is highly predictive of subsequent offending. Measures of prior offending have included the number of prior arrests (Cocozza & Steadman, 1974), prior incarcerations (Steadman & Co-cozza, 1976), arrests for disturbing the peace (Klassen & O'Conner, 1988a), previous arrests for violent crime (Thornberry & Jacoby, 1979; Steadman & Morrissey, 1982), seriousness of prior offenses (Thornberry & Jacoby, 1979), prior sex crimes (Quinsey & McGuire, 1986), and self-reports of violent incidents (Tardiff, Marzuk, Leon, & Portera, 1997; Klassen & O'Conner, 1988a).

These research findings have been translated into advice to clinicians to weigh heavily these historical factors when making their assessments of the risk of future violent behavior. In fact, the literature ranks prior history as the single most important factor for clinicians to consider. For example, Gutheil & Appelbaum (2000) note that past violence "repeatedly appears as the strongest correlate in actuarial studies of violence and related phenom-ena" (p. 68). Melton, Petrila, Poythress, and Slobogin recommend that "for assessing baseline level of risk, historical factors such as adult criminal record and delinquency history are among the most important factors that may inform clinical judgments" (1997, p. 289). Finally, McNiel concludes, "A history of violence has been consistently shown to be the best single predictor of future violent behavior" (1998, p. 96).

Another theme in much of the recent clinical literature is the willingness of patients to report violence and criminal histories when directly and ap-propriately asked. Gutheil and Appelbaum prodded clinicians in this area, noting that "Clinicians must overcome their denial based on discomfort with the issues of violence, in order to make a specific inquiry about this subject. . . . This may elicit unexpected, but highly relevant data. . . ." (2000, p. 68). McNiel believes that "Obtaining a violence history is an essential part of assessing a patient's risk of violence. Recent studies have shown a willingness of patients to self-report a history of violence that is remarkable in view of the socially undesirable nature of the behavior" (1998, p. 97). As will be evident from the data immediately following, our research reinforces these prior writings with regard to both the basic relationships and their clinical relevance.

Measures of Prior Violence and Criminality in the MacArthur Study

Several measures of prior violence and criminality are available for analysis spanning a range of data sources and time frames (see Table 3.2). *Recent violence* refers to any act of violence committed by a patient during the 2 month period preceding admission to the hospital and was measured by patient self-report. (Recent violence may or may not have resulted in official arrest.) The *type of prior arrests* and the *frequency of prior arrests* were also measured by patient self-report and cover the period of time since the patient was 15 years old. Violent behavior as a *reason for admission* was measured by review of hospital records for evidence that violent behavior toward others contributed to the current hospitalization. *Official arrests for crimes against persons* and *official arrests for crimes against property* include those occurring after age 18 years and were gathered from arrest records obtained from state law enforcement authorities.

How Much Prior Violence and Criminality Was Present?

Table 3.2 disaggregates the sample in terms of the measures described above. As shown, 16.4% of patients had engaged in at least one act of violence toward others during the 2 months before hospital admission, and 8.2% had some evidence in their hospital record that violence was a precipitating factor with regard to the hospital admission. Approximately half the patients reported having been arrested since the age of 15 years, with just over one-fifth of patients reporting prior arrests for serious crimes involving others.

TABLE 3.2. Postdischarge Violence by Prior Violence and Criminality

Prior Violence and Criminality	Sample Description		Percent Violent After Discharge	
	No.	%	First 20 Weeks	1 Year
Recent violence				
No	785	83.6	16.3***	23.9***
Yes	154	16.4	31.2	46.1
Admission reason: violent behavior				
No	862	91.8	17.7**	26.7*
Yes	77	8.2	19.9	37.7
Type of prior arrests—self-report				
No arrests	393	50.8	9.9***	16.5***
Property/ other minor	208	26.9	21.2	31.3
Violent	173	22.3	34.7	48.6
Frequency of prior arrests—self-report				
None	393	49.7	9.9***	16.5***
Once/twice	107	13.5	17.5	30.7
Three or more	290	36.8	32.0	43.3
Official arrest: crimes against person(s)				
No	737	78.5	16.0***	21.4***
Yes	202	21.5	27.7	39.1
Official arrest: crimes against property				
No	603	64.2	15.4***	23.1***
Yes	336	35.8	24.7	35.7

* p <.05 ** p <.01 *** p <.001.

Just under 37% of patients reported having been arrested three or more times since the age of 15 years. When the measure is having an official arrest record rather than a patient's self-report of having been arrested, 21.5% of the patients were found to have been arrested for crimes against other persons, and 35.8% were found to have been arrested for crimes not involving other persons.

What Was the Relation of Prior Violence and Criminality to Later Violence?

Table 3.2 also shows the relationship between prior violence and criminality and the prevalence of postdischarge violence. Clearly, prior violence and criminality are strongly associated with the postdischarge violent behavior of psychiatric patients. The pattern of results observed in Table 3.2 was maintained when the relationship between prior violence and criminality was examined for males and females and for African-Americans and whites separately, except for the following statistically significant interaction: The 43 females who had an official arrest record for crimes against persons were no more likely to become violent after discharge than were the 358 females with no such arrest records (15.2% vs. 14.0%, respectively). This compares with a rate of violence of 16.6% for the 379 males with no history of arrests for crimes against persons and the rate of violence of 32.7% for the 159 males who had been previously arrested for such crimes.

Conclusions Regarding Prior Violence and Criminality and Postdischarge Violence

The data suggest quite clearly (and not surprisingly, given the extensive research cited above) that, regardless of how the measure is obtained, prior violence and criminality are strongly associated with the postdischarge violent behavior of psychiatric patients. The lack of association between an official record of prior arrests for crimes against persons and postdischarge violent behavior among female patients may suggest that the decision of the police to arrest women for such serious crimes is more reflective of the situational dynamics surrounding particular incidents involving women (e.g., when police are attempting to resolve domestic disputes) than of an assessment of women's likelihood of committing further acts of violence (and hence the need for incapacitation in jail).

The strength and consistency of the predictive association between prior violence and criminality and postdischarge violence make obtaining a reliable estimate of past crime and violence a high clinical priority (see Chapter 5). Often, clinicians at acute psychiatric facilities do not have access to a patient's arrest record. When such records are available or easily obtained, however, they may supply the clinician with important information. Directly asking the patient about past crime and violence, whether or not it resulted in arrest, and whether or not an arrest record is available, would appear to be an essential component of violence risk assessment (Swanson, Borum, Swartz, & Hiday, 1999).

CHILDHOOD EXPERIENCES

That exposure to disruptive and abusive family environments is related to the acquisition of violent behavior is a widely recognized tenet within the behavioral sciences (Bandura, 1973; Widom, 1989a, b; Earles & Barnes, 1997). Hypothesized causal mechanisms range from modeling ("violence breeds violence") to a lack of self-control due to being unsupervised during early childhood (Sampson & Lauritsen, 1994). This association between negative family environments in childhood and adolescence and later violence is as true of people with mental disorder as it is of people without it. In a study of male psychiatric patients, for example, Yesavage Becker, Werner, Patton, Seeman, Brunsting, and Mills (1983) found subjects' reports of parental fighting with persons outside of the family to be significantly associated with violence both before hospital admission and during hospitalization. Other studies have found similar associations with subsequent arrest and rehospitalization for violence measured within 6 months and 1 year from hospital admission (Klassen & O'Conner, 1988a). Furthermore, injury from an adult received before a child is 15 years old has been found to be predictive of subsequent violence in schizophrenic and nonschizophrenic male patients (Klassen & O'Conner, 1988b), and severe paternal discipline has been found to be predictive of in-hospital violence among male schizophrenic patients (Yesavage, 1984).

Other experiences within the family environment have also been shown to affect subsequent violent behavior. For example, parental loss, whether due to death, separation, or divorce, has been found to correlate with later adult violence (Quinsey, Warneford, Pruesse, & Link, 1975; Klassen and O'Conner, 1988b, 1990; Climent, Rollins, Ervin, & Plutchik, 1973). In addition, disruption in the family environment (i.e., due to parental psychiatric hospitalizations, arrests, and/or drug and alcohol abuse) has been found to correlate with adult violence among persons with mental disorders (Convit, Jaeger, Lin, Meisner, & Volavka, 1988).

Measures of Childhood Experiences in the MacArthur Study

A significant portion of the baseline interview administered to patients in the hospital was devoted to assessing their childhood experiences. Questions focused on a range of experiences, including physical and sexual abuse, parental drug and alcohol abuse, parental arrest histories, family stability, and parental psychiatric treatment. From these questions, 15 measures were constructed (see Table 3.3).

What Were the Patients' Childhood Experiences?

As shown in Table 3.4, fully 41.1% of the patients reported having been sexually abused before age 20 years. There is a significant difference by gender, with 61.0% of the female patients reporting prior sexual abuse compared with 26.1% of the male patients. Furthermore, a large proportion of patients reported histories of serious physical childhood abuse, with 52.5% reporting having been hit with an object and 23.1% reporting having been injured to the point of requiring medical attention. Sixty-nine percent of patients reported childhood physical abuse occurring sometimes (33.3%) or frequently (35.7%) (see Rose, Peabody, & Stratigeas, 1991). There were no significant gender differences in either the frequency or the seriousness of self-reported childhood physical abuse.

In terms of parental behaviors, just over 19% of patients reported episodes of excessive drug use by the father that occurred either weekly or daily, and just over 60% reported a similar level of excessive paternal alcohol use. Approximately one-third of subjects reported that the father was arrested at least once during their childhood years, and 12.6% reported at least one psychiatric hospitalization for the father. Just under half of patients reported living with the father until age 15 years.

Mothers were less likely than fathers to be described as having used alcohol or drugs excessively on a weekly or daily basis (7.0% and 25.7%, respectively, compared with 19.1% and 61.7% for fathers). Patients were also less likely to report maternal than paternal arrests (21.2% vs. 37.8% for fathers). Approximately 17% of mothers were reported to have experienced at least one psychiatric hospitalization, slightly higher than the rate for fathers. Just over three-fourths of patients reported living with the mother until age 15 years. Just under 15% of patients described parents as fighting with each other frequently, and approximately 4% reported parents fighting frequently with others outside of the family.

TABLE 3.3. Developmental and Historical Measures

Measure	Description
Childhood sexual abuse	Self-report to the question: Did anyone ever bother you sexually or try to have sex with you against your will? (1 = any sexual abuse occurring before age 20 years; 2 = no)
Child abuse seriousness	Twelve self-report questions on the type of abuse by his or her parents that a patient experienced as a child (0 = none; 1 = bare hand only, with no physical injury; 2 = with an object, with no physical injury; 3 = resulting in physical injury)
Child abuse frequency	Twelve self-report questions on the frequency of abuse by his or her parents that a patient experienced as a child (0 = none, 1 = once/ twice, 2 = sometimes, 3 = frequently)
Father's excessive drug use	Self-report question on whether the patient's father had ever used drugs excessively (1 = weekly/daily, 0 = less often)
Father's excessive alcohol use	Self-report question on whether the patient's father had ever used alcohol excessively (1 = weekly/daily, 0 = less often)
Father arrested	Self-report question on whether the patient's father had ever been arrested or convicted of a crime (0 = never, 1 = at least once)
Father's admissions for psychiatric treatment	Self-report question on whether the patient's father had ever been admitted to a psychiatric hospital (0 = never, 1 = once/twice, 2 = several times, 3 = very often)
Lived with father	Self-report question on whether the patient had lived with the father until age 15 years (0 = no, 1 = yes)
Mother's excessive drug use	Self-report question on whether the patient's mother had ever used drugs excessively (1 = weekly/daily, 0 = less often)
Mother's excessive alcohol use	Self-report question on whether the patient's mother had ever used alcohol excessively (1 = weekly/daily, 0 = less often)
Mother arrested	Self-report question on whether the patient's mother had ever been arrested or convicted of a crime (0 = never, 1 = at least once)
Mother's admissions for psychiatric treatment	Self-report question on whether the patient's mother had ever been admitted to a psychiatric hospital (0 = never, 1 = once/twice, 2 = several times, 3 = very often)

(continued)

TABLE 3.3.—Continued

Measure	Description
Lived with mother	Self-report question on whether the patient had lived with the mother until age 15 years (0 = no 1 = yes)
Parental disputes	Self-report question on whether the patient's parents had fought with each other (0 = never, 1 = once/twice, 2 = sometimes, 3 = frequently)
Parents fought with others outside family	Self-report question on whether the patient's parents had fought with others outside of family (0 = never, 1 = once/twice, 2 = sometimes, 3 = frequently)

What Was the Relation of Childhood Experiences to Later Violence?

Table 3.4 also shows the relationship between the family experiences described above and the prevalence of postdischarge violence. A number of observations may be drawn, focusing on the 1 year prevalence of violence. First, having been sexually abused before age 20 years showed no association with post-discharge violence. This lack of association held when examined separately for males and females and for African-American and white patients. In contrast, the seriousness and frequency of prior physical abuse as a child was found to be associated with an increased rate of postdischarge violence, with the highest rates of violence observed among those who had experienced the most serious and frequent levels of childhood physical abuse. These associations did not vary by the gender or race of the patient.

Behaviors of the father during the patients' childhood were also found to be associated with violence following hospital discharge. These behaviors included fathers' excessive drug use, excessive alcohol use, and arrests for illegal conduct. In contrast, hospital admissions of the father for psychiatric treatment were not associated with post-discharge patient violence.

Despite the effects on violence of paternal drug use, alcohol use, and arrests, having lived with the father until age 15 years was associated with a *decreased* rate of violence among patients. This apparent anomaly is easily explained: The fathers who were home until the patient was 15 years old were very different from the fathers who were absent. The patients reported

TABLE 3.4. Postdischarge Violence by Childhood Family Experiences

Family Experience	Sample Description		Percent Violent After Discharge	
			First 20	
	No.	%	Weeks	1 Year
Sexually abused before Age 20 years				
No	537	58.9	19.9	28.9
Yes	374	41.1	17.4	26.2
Child abuse seriousness				
None reported	172	18.3	10.5***	17.0***
Hit with bare hand	57	6.1	7.0	15.8
Hit with object	493	52.5	19.7	29.0
Injury requiring medical attention	217	23.1	26.3	35.5
Child abuse frequency				
None reported	172	18.3	10.5***	17.4***
Once/twice	119	12.7	15.1	22.7
Sometimes	313	33.3	19.8	25.9
Frequently	335	35.7	23.3	36.1
Father's excessive drug use				
Less than once a week	691	80.9	16.4***	24.7***
Weekly or daily	163	19.1	31.9	42.3
Father's excessive alcohol use				
Less than once a week	341	38.3	13.5**	21.1***
Weekly or daily	549	61.7	22.6	32.2
Father arrested				
Never	521	62.2	14.4***	22.5***
Once	261	31.1	25.3	36.4
Two or more	56	6.7	32.1	41.1
Father's admissions for psychiatric treatment				
Never	744	87.4	18.4	27.8
Once or more	107	12.6	20.6	28.0
Lived with father until age 15 years				
No	483	51.4	22.2**	32.1**
Yes	456	48.6	15.1	22.8
Mother's excessive drug use				
Less than weekly	821	93.0	18.4	27.0*
Weekly or daily	62	7.0	25.8	40.3
Mother's excessive alcohol use				
Less than weekly	656	74.3	17.1	25.5*
Weekly or daily	227	25.7	22.5	32.6
Mother arrested				
Never	798	78.8	17.7	26.6
Once	60	6.6	23.3	31.7
Two or more	51	5.6	23.5	31.4

(continued)

TABLE 3.4.—Continued

Family Experience	Sample Description		Percent Violent After Discharge	
			First 20	
	No.	%	Weeks	1 Year
Mother's admissions for psychiatric treatment				
Never	726	83.4	19.1	28.8
Once/twice	101	11.6	18.8	25.7
Three or more	44	5.1	13.6	18.2
Lived with mother until age 15 years				
No	211	22.5	22.7	33.2*
Yes	728	77.5	17.6	26.0
Parental disputes (with each other)				
Never	525	61.8	16.6	24.0**
Once/twice	58	6.8	17.2	22.4
Sometimes	142	16.7	22.5	31.0
Frequently	124	14.6	21.0	38.7
Parents fought outside of family				
Never	680	76.2	17.9	26.3
Once/twice	79	8.9	25.3	34.2
Sometimes	96	10.8	19.8	31.3
Frequently	37	4.1	21.6	15.1

* p <.05 ** p <.01 ***p <.001.

excessive drug use for 10.2% of the fathers who were present and for 28.6% of the fathers who were absent. Excessive alcohol use was reported for 52.3% of the fathers who were present and for 71.2% of the fathers who were absent. Finally, arrests for illegal conduct were reported for 26.3% of the fathers who were present and for 50.0% of the fathers who were absent. Clearly, the fathers who remained living at home until the patients were 15 years old were much less "criminogenic" than were the fathers who had left by then.

Interestingly, the association between father's drug use and patient violence was found to interact significantly with patient race, with a much stronger association observed for white patients than for African-American patients. Specifically, the rate of violence among white patients whose fathers abused drugs (n = 104) was 57.7% compared with 19.9% who were violent among white patients whose fathers did not abuse drugs (n = 488); the rate of violence among the African-American patients whose fathers abused drugs (n = 59) was 42.4% compared with 36.5% who were violent among the African-American patients whose fathers did not abuse drugs (n = 203). Similarly, the negative association between violence and having lived with the father until age 15 years was found to be highly significant for white patients, but not for African-American patients. No differences by gender were observed in the effects on violence of prior behaviors of the father.

In terms of behaviors attributed by patients to their mothers, Table 3.4 shows a significant positive association with violence during the 1 year period following discharge for excessive maternal drinking and excessive maternal drug use. The effect of mother's excessive drug use on patient violence during this period was, however, found to interact significantly with patient gender, with all of the effect occurring for males and none of the effect occurring for females. Specifically, males who reported excessive maternal drug use (n = 38) showed a 52.6% rate of violence, compared with a rate of violence of 28.8% for males who did not report excessive maternal drug use. In contrast, female patients showed a rate of violence between 21% and 25%, regardless of excessive maternal drug use. The effect of excessive maternal alcohol use on violence did not vary by patient gender or race.

Despite the effects of maternal alcohol and drug use on violence, living with the mother until age 15 years was associated with a lower rate of violence during the 1 year period following discharge, an effect that did not vary by patient gender or race. Similar to observations for fathers, hospital admissions of the mother for psychiatric treatment were not associated with postdischarge patient violence. Finally, patients who reported a history of their parents frequently fighting with each other were significantly more likely than were patients without such a history to become violent in the 1 year postdischarge follow-up period, an effect that did not vary by gender or race of the patient.

Conclusions Regarding Childhood Experiences and Violence

Taken as a whole, the results suggest a fair amount of complexity in the associations between childhood family experiences and postdischarge violent behavior among psychiatric patients. Although prior physical abuse as a child was associated with postdischarge violence, prior sexual abuse was not. Although patients' reports of deviant behaviors by fathers and mothers, such as excessive alcohol and drug use (and arrests for fathers only), were associated with increased rates of postdischarge violence, having lived with either the father or the mother before age 15 years was associated with a decreased rate of violence. Furthermore, the increased risk for violence associated with paternal drug use was found to be stronger for white patients than for African-American patients, the increased risk for violence associated with maternal drug use was found to be limited to male patients, and the decreased risk for violence associated with living with the father until age 15 years was found to be limited to white patients.

These findings demonstrate both the general importance of childhood experiences as risk factors for postdischarge violence and the contingency of the relationships between specific experiences and later violence. Some childhood experiences, such as having been seriously physically abused, raise the rates of subsequent violence across the board, regardless of a patient's demographic characteristics. Other childhood experiences, however, such as a father's or a mother's drug use, have a violence-enhancing effect that appears to be specific to one gender or racial group. The conditional nature of many of these observed relationships led us to focus in subsequent chapters of this book on developing a violence risk assessment procedure that is based on interactions among risk factors rather than on across-the-board main effects.

NEIGHBORHOOD

In recent years, there has been a surge of interest in neighborhood risk and protective factors for violence in the field of criminology (Sampson, Raudenbush, & Earls, 1997). This research shows that residents of socioeconomically disadvantaged, socially isolated neighborhoods are more likely to engage in violence (Anderson, 1990; Land, McCall, & Cohen, 1990) and to become the victims of violent crime (Miethe & McDowall, 1993). With rare exceptions (e.g., Estroff & Zimmer, 1994; Hiday, 1995), however, studies of the violent behavior of persons with mental illness have focused exclusively on the explanatory power of individual-level variables. This is due, in part, to the difficulty of collecting relevant social context measures—particularly when an individual is evaluated in a clinical setting, outside his or her usual social context—and, in part, to the belief that violence risk is largely individually determined. In contrast, a focus on neighborhood risk factors emphasizes social and situational experiences that may, in conjunction with individual characteristics, influence the occurrence of violent behavior among persons with mental disorder.

Silver, Mulvey, and Monahan (1999), using data from the MacArthur Violence Risk Assessment Study, found that patients who resided in high-poverty census tracts following discharge from Pittsburgh's Western Psychiatric Institute and Clinic (WPIC) were more likely to engage in violence than were patients discharged into lower poverty neighborhoods. This result held after key individual characteristics, such as gender, age, race, socioeconomic status, substance abuse disorder, and psychopathy, were taken into account. In addition, the socioeconomic status of individual patients was found to be less predictive of violent behavior than was concentrated poverty in the neighborhood.

This finding is important for two reasons. First, it demonstrates the significant independent effect of concentrated poverty on violence by discharged psychiatric patients, holding constant other important risk factors. Second, it addresses the concern that the observed neighborhood effect is due primarily to neighborhood selection factors occurring at hospital discharge. If the observed neighborhood effect was due to the systematic discharge of more potentially violent patients to neighborhoods with more concentrated poverty, then controlling for factors related to perceived dangerousness, such as gender, age, race, socioeconomic status, substance abuse disorder, and psychopathy, would have "explained away" the concentrated poverty effect. That these individual characteristics did not explain away the neighborhood effect suggests that the effect of concentrated poverty on violence is not an artifact related to the systematic assignment of more dangerous patients to higher poverty neighborhoods.

Here, we provide a brief, but dramatic, example that further underscores the importance of contextual measurement in violence risk assessment research. Our example features the joint effects of race and neighborhood disadvantage on violence among the patients treated at WPIC. This analysis is guided by a considerable amount of criminological research on non-mentally ill populations indicating that (1) rates of violent behavior are significantly higher among African-Americans; (2) rates of violent behavior are significantly higher in neighborhoods that are socioeconomically disadvantaged; and (3) African-Americans are significantly more likely to reside in socioeconomically disadvantaged neighborhoods (Sampson & Lauritsen, 1994). Taken together, these findings indicate that individual-level associations between racial status and violent behavior may be systematically confounded with levels of disadvantage in the neighborhood contexts of African-Americans. This possibility suggests that empirical assessments of the relationship between minority racial status and violent behavior take into account the neighborhood contexts within which minority individuals reside.

Measures of Neighborhood Context in the MacArthur Study

A shortcoming of the analysis reported by Silver et al. (1999) was that only a single measure was used to represent the extent of socioeconomic disadvantage in the neighborhoods in which patients resided following hospital discharge (i.e., neighborhood poverty). In contrast, the analysis reported here uses a more sophisticated measure of neighborhood context by constructing a neighborhood disadvantage factor score from a wide range of measures known to be related to neighborhood disadvantage, including neighborhood poverty, neighborhood income, the extent of female-headed families in the neighborhood, neighborhood employment rates and occupational structure, neighborhood residential stability, and the quality of neighborhood housing stock. (Silver [2000, in press] describes the factor analytic techniques used to combine these measures into a single neighborhood disadvantage factor score.) Neighborhood racial composition was not included in the list of neighborhood measures to avoid confounding the neighborhood disadvantage score with patients' racial status. The neighborhood disadvantage factor score was linked to the patient data set by using census tract identifiers corresponding to the addresses at which patients resided following treatment at WPIC.

What Was the Relation of Neighborhood Context to Violence?

Due to the small number of Hispanic patients treated at WPIC, only white and African-American patients were included in the analysis. We examine acts of violence, coded as a dichotomous measure, that occurred during the first 20 weeks following discharge from WPIC. Although data on violence were gathered over a 1 year period, we focus on a 20 week period here because it is for this period that the census tract locations of patients were known. Assessments of contextual effects beyond this period are problematic as subjects are likely to change residences, thereby jeopardizing the validity of the contextual measure.

Part A of Table 3.5 displays the significant bivariate association between African-American race and community violence. The remaining parts of Table 3.5, however, show that when the sample is disaggregated in terms of the levels of disadvantage in the neighborhoods in which patients resided, the significant association between race and violence disappears. That is, despite the overall association between race and violence in this sample, African Americans and whites residing in comparably disadvantaged neighborhoods showed no differences in their rates of violence.

The reason we observed a significant association between African-American racial status and violence in the full sample is that African-American patients were more likely to reside in disadvantaged neighborhoods where all patients, regardless of race, were more likely to become violent. This result was confirmed when we examined it with a logistic regression model predicting the occurrence of violence: The significant odds ratio for African-American racial status (odds ratio = 2.7) was significantly attenuated (odds ratio = 1.3) when neighborhood disadvantage was added

TABLE 3.5. Postdischarge Violence by Race and Neighborhood Disadvantage

Neighborhood Description	Patient Race	% Violent
A. All neighborhoods (33.7% African American)	African American (n = 91) White (n = 179)	19.8** 8.4
B. Low disadvantage neighborhoods (4.4% African American)	African American (n = 4) White (n = 86)	0.0 3.5
C. Medium disadvantage neighborhoods (27.2% African American)	African American (n = 31) White (n = 83)	12.9 12.0
D. High disadvantage neighborhoods (84.8% African American)	African American (n = 56) White (n = 10)	25.0 20.0

** $p < .01$.

to the equation. The effect of neighborhood disadvantage, however, remained significant (odds ratio = 1.7).

In this study, as with all research aimed at relating contextual factors to individual-level outcomes, the problem of selection bias must always be considered as an alternative interpretation. Our confidence in this particular analysis is increased to the extent that the neighborhoods in which patients resided after discharge were the same as the neighborhoods where they lived before admission to the hospital. If, in contrast, subjects who were prone to violence were systematically relocated to disadvantaged neighborhoods, our confidence in these findings would be diminished.

To address this potential confound, we compared patients' postdischarge census tracts with their zip code areas before admission to the hospital. We found that, of the 270 subjects in this study, 207 (76.7%) were discharged into census tracts within the zip code area of the preadmission address. This high rate of subjects discharged into the same zip code area from which they came lends credence to our interpretation of the effect of neighborhood disadvantage as a contextual effect that is not due to selection processes operating from within the hospital. Our confidence is further bolstered by the observation that 80.3% of subjects were living at home (i.e., in a private house or apartment) at the time of their first follow-up interview in the community (approximately 10 weeks from the date of discharge) rather than on the street or in a half-way house. Thus, the likelihood that patients had been reassigned to neighborhoods by hospital staff is not supported by the data.

Conclusions Regarding Neighborhood Context and Violence

The results of this analysis suggest that studies of violence among persons with mental illness that include individual-level predictors—of which race is only one illustration—but do not control for such contextual measures as neighborhood disadvantage run the risk of overstating the effect of the individual-level variables. Indeed, part of the reason for the lack of consistency found in prior studies of the relationship between race and violence among discharged patients (Klassen & O'Conner, 1994) may relate to differences in the neighborhood contexts of the samples studied.

This analysis demonstrates the utility of employing a contextual approach to the problem of assessing violence risk among persons discharged from a psychiatric hospital. The findings suggest that research efforts aimed at assessing violence risk among discharged psychiatric patients may benefit from specifying a role for the neighborhood contexts into which patients are discharged, in addition to measuring their individual characteristics. These findings also suggest that violence by persons with mental disorders may be, in part, a function of the high-crime neighborhoods in which they typically reside. To the extent that this is true, these findings raise important questions about the locations of half-way houses and other living facilities for the mentally ill. One part of an overall strategy for reducing violence may be to locate such facilities in less disadvantaged, lower crime neighborhoods.

The clinical implications of these findings lie in emphasizing the importance of assessing contextual conditions, as well as individual characteristics, when predicting and managing the risk for violence posed by discharged patients. Specifically, the findings reported here suggest that one important, albeit partial, way to manage risk for violence among psychiatric patients may be to focus on the neighborhood environments into which patients are being discharged in addition to their psychiatric conditions at the time of discharge. Of course, the findings reported here and by Silver et al. (1999) indicate that individual characteristics are also essential in the assessment and management of violence risk, as these explain a significant proportion of variation in violent outcomes.

CONCLUSIONS

We believe that the complexity of the results found here testing key "criminological" variables reflects the difficulty of identifying across-the-board risk factors for violence in all people with mental disorder. These results counsel the adoption of an *interactional* approach to violence risk assessment rather than one that relies on "main effects" that apply uniformly to all patients. We elaborate on this point at the conclusion of the following chapter, which highlights a number of clinical risk factors.

4

TESTING "CLINICAL" RISK FACTORS

As mentioned earlier, advice to clinicians on how to assess violence risk has usually consisted of emphasizing a set of "key" risk factors that clinicians are admonished to take into account when making predictive judgments. The MacArthur Violence Risk Assessment Study provided an opportunity to test the relationships between a large number of these proffered risk factors and subsequent violence. The previous chapter considered risk factors taken from the "criminological" tradition — gender, prior violence and criminality, childhood experiences, and neighborhood. In this chapter, we address more "clinical" variables of diagnosis, psychopathy, delusions, hallucinations, violent thoughts, and anger.

DIAGNOSIS

Much clinical lore attests to the relationship between a diagnosis of schizophrenia and the occurrence of violence. Popular belief is along much the same lines: 61% of the American population believe that people with schizophrenia are "very" or "somewhat" likely "to do something violent to others" (Pescosolido, Monahan, Link, Stueve, & Kikuzawa, 1999). In fact, however, the relationship between diagnosis and violence has long been confusing and contested.

Some investigators have found that people with schizophrenia have higher rates of violence than people with other Axis I diagnoses (Baxter, 1997). Others have found that women with schizophrenia have higher rates of violence than women with other diagnoses, but men with schizophrenia do not (Wessely, 1997). Still others have found people with schizophrenia to have *lower* rates of violence than people with other Axis I diagnoses (Gardner, Lidz, Mulvey, & Shaw, 1996b; Tiihonen, Isohanni, Rasanen, Koiranen, & Moring, 1997). There are also investigators who have found no difference in the rate of violence across Axis I categories of major mental disorder (Swanson, Holzer, Gunju, & Jono, 1990; Belfrage, 1998). In addition, some researchers have found that the highest rates of violence are not among Axis I diagnoses at all, but rather among Axis II diagnoses (Rice & Harris, 1995a; Tardiff, Marzuk, Leon, & Portera, 1997; Wallace, Mullen, Burgess, Palmer, Ruschena, & Brown,1998). Many studies do not address the "compared to whom?" issue. For example, people with the diagnosis of schizophrenia may have a lower rate of violence than people with an Axis II diagnosis, but a higher rate of violence than people with no diagnosis at all. Adding to this muddle, many of the relevant studies have been conducted in Scandinavia, and, as Tiihonen et al. (1997) note, these studies "may be generalizable to other industrialized Western countries that have relatively low crime rates (e.g., Sweden, Denmark, Norway, United Kingdom, and Canada) but not to countries with high crime rates such as the United States" (p. 844).

What were the Patients' Diagnoses in the MacArthur Study?

A research clinician (Ph.D. or MA/MSW) confirmed the chart diagnosis using the DSM-III-R Checklist (Janca & Helzer, 1990) or confirmed a personality disorder using the Structured Interview for DSM-III-R Personality (Pfohl, Blum, Zimmerman, & Stangl, 1989) when no eligible Axis I diagnosis was present. Checklist diagnoses corresponded to a chart diagnosis in 85.7% of the cases. Discrepant diagnoses were resolved by a consultant psychiatrist at each site.

As noted in Appendix A, depression was the most frequent primary research diagnosis (41.9%), followed by Alcohol/Drug Abuse/Dependence (21.8%), Schizophrenia (17.0%), Bipolar Disorder (14.1%), Personality Disorder Only (2.1%), and Other Psychotic Disorder (3.1%). The proportion of all cases with a primary research diagnosis of major mental disorder—see the following paragraph for the specific diagnoses included—that had a co-occurring diagnosis of substance abuse or dependence was as follows: Depression, 49.6%; Schizophrenia, 41.0%; Bipolar Disorder, 37.7%; and Other Psychotic Disorder, 45.0%.

What Was the Relation of Diagnosis to Violence?

Rates of violence were calculated separately for three broad diagnostic groups, as determined by our research clinicians (for a full description of these results, see Steadman et al., 1998). The first group (n = 395 for the first 20 weeks and 397 for the 1 year aggregate) consisted of patients with a diagnosis of major mental disorder—Schizophrenia, Schizophreniform, Schizoaffective, Depression, Dysthymia, Mania, Cyclothymia, or Other Psychotic Disorder (including Delusional Disorder, Atypical Psychosis, and Brief Reactive Psychosis)—who did not also have a diagnosis of substance abuse or dependence (the Major Mental Disorder/No Substance Abuse group). The second group (n = 386 for the first 20 weeks and 392 for the 1 year aggregate) consisted of patients with a diagnosis of major mental disorder and a co-occurring diagnosis of substance abuse/dependence (the Major Mental Disorder/Substance Abuse group).[1] The third group (n = 138 for the first 20 weeks and 142 for the 1 year aggregate) consisted of patients with a diagnosis of an "other" mental disorder (i.e., a personality or an adjustment disorder and several cases of "suicidality") and a co-occurring diagnosis of substance abuse/dependence (the Other Mental Disorder/Substance Abuse group).

We found a 1 year rate of violence for the Major Mental Disorder/No Substance Abuse group of 17.9%. The co-occurrence of substance abuse clearly elevates the rate of violence: the Major Mental Disorder/Substance Abuse group had a 1 year prevalence rate of 31.1%. Even this, however, was exceeded by the Other Mental Disorder/Substance Abuse group, which demonstrated a rate of 43.0% (Table 4.1). The corresponding rates for the

---

[1] Patients in either of the Major Mental Disorder groups may and often did have co-occurring Axis II diagnoses, which are not analyzed here.

TABLE 4.1. Prevalence of Violence (%) by Broad Diagnostic Groups

	Major Mental Disorder, No Substance Abuse	Major Mental Disorder and Substance Abuse	Other Mental Disorder and Substance Abuse	Total Sample
First 20 weeks	10.1	22.3	32.6	18.7***
1 Year	17.9	31.1	43.0	27.5***

*** p <.001.

first 20 weeks after discharge were 10.1%, 22.3%, and 32.6%, respectively. Analyses revealed significant main effects on violence for diagnostic group for the 1 year aggregate and for the first 20 weeks.

The Major Mental Disorder group consisted primarily of patients who had a diagnosis of Schizophrenia (n = 160 for the first 20 weeks and 162 for the 1 year aggregate), Major Depression (n = 393 for the first 20 weeks and 397 for the 1 year aggregate), or Bipolar Disorder (n = 132 for both the first 20 weeks and the 1 year aggregate).

Contrary to the public view that people with schizophrenia are much more likely to be violent than are people with depression (Pescosolido, Monahan, Link, Stueve, & Kikuzawa, 1999), the 1 year prevalence rate of violence was 14.8% for patients with schizophrenia, 28.5% for patients with depression, and 22.0% for patients with bipolar disorder, a statistically significant difference. The corresponding violence rates for the first 20 weeks postdischarge were 8.1% for patients with schizophrenia, 18.8% for patients with depression, and 15.2% for patients with bipolar disorder, a difference that was also statistically significant. Among patients who had a primary research diagnosis of one of the three major mental disorders described above, the presence of a co-occurring diagnosis of alcohol or drug abuse or dependence was significantly related to violence: 10.0% of the patients without co-occurring substance abuse were violent during the first 20 weeks after discharge compared with 22.5% of the patients with a co-occurring diagnosis (the figures for the 1 year follow-up period are 18.1% and 31.3%, respectively).

Conclusions Regarding Diagnosis

Confirming the findings of others (Swanson, Borum, Swartz, & Monahan, 1996; Swartz, Swanson, Hiday, Borum, Wagner, & Burns, 1998; Arseneault, Moffitt, Caspi, Taylor, & Silva, 2000), we found the presence of a co-occurring diagnosis of substance abuse or dependence to be a key factor in the occurrence of violence. Confirming still others (Lidz et al., 1993; Quinsey et al., 1998), we found that a diagnosis of a major mental disorder was associated with a lower rate of violence than was a diagnosis of an "other" mental disorder, primarily a personality or adjustment disorder. Furthermore, within the major mental disorders, a diagnosis of schizophrenia was associated with lower rates of violence than was a diagnosis of depression or of bipolar disorder. Our findings underscore the inappropriateness of referring to "discharged mental patients" as a homogeneous class regarding violence in the community.

PSYCHOPATHY[2]

Scholarly work on psychopathy has been building considerable momentum over the past decade, with a construct now considered to exist that has an "unparalleled" ability to predict future violence in criminal samples (Salekin, Rogers, & Sewell, 1996; see also Hare, 1996; Hemphill, Templeman, Wong, & Hare, 1998; Blackburn, 1998). Much of the empirical work fueling this momentum has been based on the original or revised Hare Psychopathy Checklist (Hare PCL, PCL-R; Hare, 1980, 1991) and has focused on men involved in the criminal justice system, either as prisoners or forensic psychiatric patients (see Hart, 1998a,b). These studies suggest that the PCL and the PCL-R are relatively strong predictors of general and violent recidivism among prison inmates (e.g., Hart, Kropp, & Hare, 1988; Serin & Amos, 1995) and mentally disordered offenders (e.g., Harris et al, 1993; Heilbrun, Hart, Hare, Gustafson, Nunez, & White, 1998; Rice & Harris, 1997).

Few studies, however, have investigated the Hare PCL/PCL-R in civil psychiatric samples. In response to this lack of information, Hart, Cox and

---

[2] This chapter section was co-authored by Jennifer L. Skeem, Ph.D.

Hare (1995a) developed a relatively short, screening version of the PCL (the Hare PCL:SV) to assess for psychopathy in noncriminal samples and to screen for psychopathy in criminal samples. Although normed on civil psychiatric samples, this instrument has been shown to have psychometric characteristics and total scores (r = 0.80) highly associated with those of the Hare PCL-R (Hart et al., 1995b).

There has been limited work on the predictive validity of the Hare PCL: SV. The Hare PCL:SV has been shown to predict postrelease violence among forensic psychiatric patients (Hill, Rogers, & Bickford, 1996; Strand, Belfrage, Fransson, & Levander, 1999) and to differentiate between highly select groups of psychotic patients with and without histories of persistent violent behavior (Nolan, Volavka, Mohr, & Czobor, 1999). Nevertheless, there appears to be only one published study that assesses the Hare PCL: SV's ability to predict violence among civil psychiatric patients. Using a postdictive design, Douglas et al. (1999) reviewed the files of 193 involuntarily civilly committed patients, assigned scores on the Hare PCL:SV, and assessed the measure's ability to predict postrelease community violence over an average 2 year period. Following discharge, patients who scored at or above the Hare PCL:SV sample median of 8 were 5 times more likely to commit a physically violent act and 14 times more likely to be arrested for a violent crime than were those who scored below the median.

Measure of Psychopathy in the MacArthur Study

Like its parent measures (Hare et al., 1990; Harpur, Hare, & Hakistan, 1989), the Hare PCL:SV structures clinical interviews and consolidates collateral information to assess two strongly correlated factors that are interpreted as a single construct. Factor 1 items reflect the interpersonal and affective core of psychopathy, or the "selfish, callous and remorseless use of others" (Harpur, Hakistan, & Hare, 1988; Hart et al., 1995b). Hare PCL:SV factor 1 items include *superficial, grandiose, deceitful, lacks remorse, lacks empathy,* and *doesn't accept responsibility.* Factor 2 items describe a collection of socially deviant behaviors, or a "chronically unstable and antisocial lifestyle." Hare PCL:SV factor 2 items include *impulsive, poor behavioral controls, lacks goals, irresponsible, adolescent antisocial behavior,* and *adult antisocial be-*

havior. Factors 1 and 2 can be labeled "emotional detachment" and "antisocial behavior," respectively (after Patrick, Bradley, & Lang, 1993).

What Proportion of Patients Were Potentially Psychopaths?

The Hare PCL:SV provides categorical as well as dimensional measures of psychopathy. Hart et al. (1995b) chose cutting scores for the categorical measures based on their efficiency in predicting PCL-R psychopathy classifications: Scores of 12 or less indicate nonpsychopathy, whereas scores of 13 to 17 indicate potential psychopathy, and scores of 18 or more strongly suggest psychopathy. Applying the threshold for probable psychopathy (18 or above) of Hart et al. (1995), the prevalence of psychopathy among civil patients in this study is only 8%, in keeping with past research (Hart et al., 1995b). This base rate is roughly three times lower than the rates found in forensic and correctional samples (Hart et al., 1995b; Hare, 1998). Given the low base rate of probable psychopathy in this sample, the categorical measure of psychopathy used in these analyses classifies study participants as "nonpsychopathic" (scores $\leq$ 12; 78% of the sample) or "potentially psychopathic" (scores $>$ 12; 22% of the sample).

What Was the Relation of Psychopathy to Violence?

Treating psychopathy as a categorical measure, we found that the relationship between the Hare PCL:SV and violence generalizes beyond criminal samples to civil psychiatric patients. (A full account of these analyses can be found in Skeem and Mulvey [in press a].) As shown in Table 4.2, the prevalence of violence was significantly lower for the "nonpsychopathic" patients than for the "potentially psychopathic" patients during both the first 20 weeks after discharge ($\chi^2[1, n = 860] = 60.01, p = .000$) and the entire 1 year follow-up period ($\chi^2[1, n = 871] = 58.07, p = .000$). In the remainder of this section, the measure of violence used is based on the full 1 year follow-up period because psychopathy is a relatively stable construct (Harpur & Hare, 1994; Lynam, 1996), and violence risk associated with psychopathy should not fluctuate across even a long follow-up interval.

The dimensional nature of the relationship between Hare PCL:SV *total*

TABLE 4.2. Hare PCL:SV Classification and the Frequency of Postdischarge Violence

	% Violent	
Psychopathy	First 20 Weeks	1 Year
Nonpsychopathic participants	13.0 (n = 87)***	21.9 (n = 148)***
Potentially psychopathic participants	37.7 (n = 72)	49.7 (n = 97)

*** p <.001.

scores and violence during the year after discharge was determined by using receiver operating characteristic (ROC) analyses (see Chapter 5). The area under the ROC curve (AUC) in this analysis was .73, indicating that there is a 73% chance that a patient who becomes violent will obtain a higher score on the Hare PCL:SV than will a randomly chosen patient who does not become violent.

Like Douglas et al. (1999), we found, using ROC analyses, that a Hare PCL:SV threshold score of approximately 8 simultaneously balances both the sensitivity (0.72) and specificity (0.65) of the Hare PCL:SV in predicting violence. That is, civil patients who obtain total Hare PCL:SV scores of 8 or above are more likely to become involved in violence than are those whose scores are below 8. This threshold for maximally predicting violence is considerably lower than the Hare PCL:SV scores suggested for diagnosing psychopathy (18) and potential psychopathy (13) (Hart et al., 1995b). Thus, civil psychiatric patients with several *traits* of psychopathy or *features* of antisocial behavior are at greater risk for violence than are those without, even if they fail to meet Hare PCL:SV diagnostic thresholds.

Some critics, however, believe that the predictive power of the PCL measures is based not on their measurement of a unique personality construct but on their systematic "packaging" of nonspecific behavioral predictors of violence, such as criminal history. Toch (1998), for example, argues that the PCL measures' predictive power is based on the principle that the "best predictor of future misbehavior is past misbehavior — especially if the misbehavior is habitual and the miscreant is young . . ." (p. 150).

A few groups (Harris, Rice, & Cormier, 1991; Hart et al., 1988; Heilbrun et al., 1998; Rice, Harris, & Quinsey, 1990) have begun to address this issue in criminal samples by assessing the relationship between the PCL/PCL-R and violence after deleting PCL items that reflect criminal history or statistically controlling for gross indices of criminal history and demographic characteristics. These studies indicate that the predictive validity of the PCL/ PCL-R total scores is not solely attributable to variables such as arrest history, gender, or age. Only rarely, however, have these studies controlled for critical variables related to psychopathy and violence among the mentally ill, such as substance abuse (cf. Hill et al., 1996). Moreover, they have not used civil psychiatric samples.

We conducted a rigorous test of the incremental validity of the Hare PCL: SV in civil psychiatric samples by identifying the chief correlates of the Hare PCL:SV and violence, statistically removing their effect, then testing the Hare PCL:SV's unique effect in predicting violence. The 15 covariates that we controlled for consisted of (1) criminal and violence history (frequency of prior arrests; arrests for crimes against persons; arrests for crimes against property; recent violence); (2) substance use and diagnosis (any alcohol-or drug-related diagnosis; any drug use during the study); (3) other personality disorders (antisocial, or "Cluster B" personality disorder); (4) anger (the Behavioral subscale of the Novaco Anger Scale, described later in this chapter); and (5) demographic characteristics (gender, race, socioeconomic status, education, estimated verbal IQ). A sequential stepwise logistic regression analysis was performed to assess the incremental validity of Hare PCL:SV classifications of patients as "nonpsychopathic" and "potentially psychopathic" in predicting violence after these 15 covariates were controlled (for details, see Skeem & Mulvey [in press a]). Although the covariates alone predicted violence well the addition of participants' Hare PCL:SV classification significantly increased the predictive power of the model. Thus, the Hare PCL:SV's predictive power does not appear to be based solely on the extent to which it reflects past criminal and violent acts, substance abuse, personality disorders other than psychopathy, or "high risk" demographic characteristics.

Hare and his colleagues believe that psychopathy is defined by the joint presence of "emotional detachment" and "antisocial behavior," the two related factors of the PCL measures (e.g., Hare, 1999). Lilienfeld (1994, 1998), however, has cogently argued that the two-factor model does not define psychopathy as much as embody a major, ongoing debate "about the primacy of and relationship between two constructs that are consistently distinguished in the literature" (Pilkonis & Klein, 1997, p. 109; see also Widiger et al., 1996). The "personality-based" model (Lilienfeld, 1994, 1998), exemplified by Cleckley's seminal work (1941), focuses on a core cluster of personality traits that roughly correspond to the PCL "emotional detachment" factor. In contrast, the "behavior-based approach" (Robins, 1966) emphasizes a long history of observable socially deviant behaviors, including those tapped by the PCL "antisocial behavior" factor.

Because the factor scores of the PCL measures "permit the social deviance component of psychopathy to be separated from the cluster of personality traits that are fundamental to the construct" (Hare, Harpur, Hakistan, Forth, Hart, & Newman, 1990, p. 340), we used them to test these views. We found that the power of the Hare PCL:SV in predicting violence in civil psychiatric samples has relatively little to do with personality traits of psychopathy, as traditionally construed (i.e., those of the "emotional detachment" factor). First, patients' scores on the "antisocial behavior" factor predicted violence more strongly (n = 0.38) than their scores on the "emotional detachment" factor (n = 0.28). In addition, patient's "antisocial behavior" factor scores were as predictive of violence (AUC = 0.74) as were their Hare PCL:SV total scores (AUC = 0.73), suggesting that the "emotional detachment" factor has relatively little additive effect (see Douglas et al., 1999; Harpur, Hare, & Hakistan, 1989; Hemphill & Hare, 1999; Salekin et al., 1996).

Second, and more importantly, the "antisocial behavior" factor, but *not* the "emotional detachment" factor, added incremental validity to the 15 covariates described earlier in predicting violence. A sequential stepwise logistic regression analysis (Tabachnick & Fidell, 1996) was performed by entering the Hare PCL:SV factor scores after controlling for the covariates of the Hare PCL:SV and violence (for details, see Skeem and Mulvey [in press a]). Only the "antisocial behavior" factor entered the model and significantly improved violence prediction. This is remarkable because all of the covariates were more strongly correlated with the "antisocial behavior" factor than with the "emotional detachment" factor. Despite the fact that removing their effect should have tipped the scales in favor of the core interpersonal and affective traits of psychopathy showing an effect, only the "antisocial behavior" factor added some explanatory power above that of the covariates.

Conclusions Regarding Psychopathy and Violence

The results show that the Hare PCL:SV is a strong predictor of violence in this sample; in fact, it was the strongest predictor of those tested in the study (see Chapter 5). Despite the low base rate of Hare PCL:SV psychopathy per se among these civil psychiatric patients, limited traits of psychopathy and antisocial behavior were predictive of future violence. The Hare PCL:SV added incremental validity to a host of covariates in predicting violence, including recent violence, criminal history, substance abuse, and other personality disorders. Most of the Hare PCL:SV's basic *and* unique predictive power is, however, based on its "antisocial behavior" factor rather than on its "emotional detachment" factor, which distills the core interpersonal and affective traits of psychopathy.

These latter results have implications for both future research and clinical practice. The results underscore the fact that the two-factor model underlying the PCL measures "leaves some major questions unanswered (Lilienfeld, 1994, p. 28). In response to such concerns, Cooke and Michie (in press) recently reanalyzed several large data sets to develop a three-factor model of psychopathy. This model divides the original "emotional detachment" factor into (1) an "arrogant and deceitful interpersonal style" and (2) a "deficient affective experience" factor. It also deletes several nonspecific behavioral items (e.g., adult antisocial behavior) that were found to be poor indicators of psychopathy from the original "antisocial behavior" factor to create (3) an "impulsive and irresponsible behavioral style" factor. Future work will determine the extent to which this three-factor model fits the data in this study and will examine the relative power of the three factors in predicting violence.

The existing results, however, indicate that the traditional conceptualization of the PCL "antisocial behavior" factor as representative of a socially deviant lifestyle may be misplaced, at least when the PCL measures are used with civil psychiatric patients. This factor may be tapping personality traits associated with antisocial behavior and violence rather than merely a history of behavioral deviance. Half of the items comprising the "antisocial behavior" factor relate to personality traits, including impulsivity, irresponsibility, and a lack of goals/planning. This factor may represent a personality construct that is related to violence, but not the one commonly understood as psychopathy (i.e., callousness, lack of remorse, superficiality). Thus, caution is called for when the Hare PCL:SV is used as a risk indicator (Blackburn, 1988; Gunn, 1998; Lösel, 1998). Clinicians must specifically interpret the meaning of a patient's high but subthreshold score on a PCL measure. A high score does not necessarily indicate "psychopathy" per se, particularly if the score falls below diagnostic cut-offs. Clinicians should attend to the PCL measures' two-factor structure and consistently describe the extent to which PCL scores and their effects are based on traits of "emotional detachment" or "antisocial behavior." This study suggests that civil psychiatric patients may pose greater or lesser risk, depending on the extent to which their total scores reflect "antisocial behavior" or "emotional detachment" (see Salekin et al., 1996). Total scores that predominately reflect high scores on the "antisocial behavior" items may indicate greater risk for violence than those based on high "emotional detachment" scores (see Rogers, 1995).

DELUSIONS

Delusions and violence have long been linked in the minds of both lay people and mental health professionals. Indeed, in the popular media, the prototypical dangerous mental patient is driven by "crazy ideas," often stoked by hallucinated voices, to commit an unspeakable act of violence (Berger & Gross, 1998; Grunwald & Boodman, 1998). The professional literature has numerous case reports detailing the link between delusions and violence. Even though systematic studies of forensic and civil patient populations have confirmed that most violence perpetrated by psychotic persons is *not* motivated by delusions, a substantial minority of their violent acts appears to stem from their delusional thoughts (Humphreys, Johnstone, MacMillan, & Taylor, 1992; Junginger, Parks-Levy, & McGuire, 1998; Martell & Dietz, 1992; Taylor, 1985; Virkkunen, 1974).

Although no one would quarrel with the conclusion that violence may be precipitated by delusions, these studies fail to address the question of whether delusional persons are more violent than other persons with or without mental illness. It is possible, for example, that persons with delusions may be less likely to commit violent acts for other reasons (e.g., instrumental violence). Two recent series of investigations, however, have addressed exactly this issue. Link and colleagues, drawing data from epidemiological studies in New York and Israel, identified a set of delusional symptoms — called "threat/control override (TCO)" delusions — as entirely responsible for the increased rate of violence they found among psychiatric patients and former patients compared with the nonpatients in their sample (Link et al., 1992; Link & Stueve, 1994; Link, Monahan, Stueve, & Cullen, 1999b). Subjects in Link's studies were scored as having TCO delusions if they reported ever having beliefs that there were people seeking to harm them ("threat") or that outside forces were in control of their minds ("control override"). Swanson and colleagues, reanalyzing data from the Epidemiologic Catchment Area study, supported these findings (Swanson et al., 1996). Given the importance of these initial investigations, we used the data from the MacArthur Violence Risk Assessment Study to test the TCO hypothesis.

Measures of Delusions in the MacArthur Study

To determine whether subjects were delusional, at baseline and during each follow-up interview a set of questions taken mostly from the Diagnostic Interview Schedule (DIS) was administered, for example, "In the past two months, have you believed that people were spying on you? . . . that you were under the control of some person, power or force? . . . that you had special gifts or powers?"(Robins, Helzer, Croughan, Williams, & Spitzer, 1981). Interviewers were then asked to judge, using the DSM-III-R definition of delusion, on the basis of all information available to them, whether the subjects were possibly or definitely delusional or whether the response reflected reality (e.g., drug dealers on the subject's front steps really were watching ["spying on"] him) or some other nondelusional perception (e.g., subject's expressed belief that someone was trying to "control" her was based on ex-husband's withholding of child support payments). To ensure the consistency of these determinations, a psychiatrist (P.S.A.) reviewed all of the screening forms, which contained the subjects' verbatim descriptions of their beliefs, and, when necessary, listened to audiotapes of the interviews. In only one case was the decision made to change the interviewer's scoring by moving a subject from the delusional to the nondelusional group.

At baseline, 28.9% of the sample (n = 328) manifested delusions. Subjects who were delusional received a more detailed assessment of the delusion that they identified as having the greatest recent impact on their lives. (In some cases, the interviewer had to make this choice when the subject could not.) The assessment was conducted with the MacArthur-Maudsley Delusions Assessment Scale (MMDAS), an adaptation of the Maudsley Assessment of Delusions Scale (Taylor, Garety, Buchanan, Reed, Wessely, Ray, Dunn, & Grubin, 1994), that generates scores on six noncontent-related dimensions: conviction, negative affect, acting on belief, refraining from acting because of belief, preoccupation, and pervasiveness. Further details and psychometric data on the MMDAS have been published elsewhere (Appelbaum, Robbins, & Roth, 1999).

What Was the Relation of Delusions to Violence?

As can be seen in part A of Table 4.3, delusions at baseline did not have a significant relationship with violence during the first 20 weeks, but did have a weakly significant *negative* relationship with violence over the entire year of follow up ($\chi^2 = 4.12$, df = 1, p = .04). That is, subjects who were delusional in the hospital were *less* likely to be violent after discharge. When different types of delusions were examined separately, this significant negative relationship was found both during the first 20 weeks and over the entire year for persecutory delusions and delusions of body/mind control (although

TABLE 4.3. Delusions Prior to Hospitalization and Postdischarge Violence

	% Violent	
Delusions	First 20 Weeks	1 Year
A. Any Delusions		
No	20.0 (n = 135)	29.4 (n = 201)*
Yes	15.5 (n = 41)	22.8 (n = 61)
B. TCO Delusions		
No	20.4 (n = 155)**	29.4 (n = 226)**
Yes	11.7 (n = 21)	19.7 (n = 36)

TCO = Threat/control override.

* p = .05 ** p = .01.

both would have been expected to predict violence according to the TCO hypothesis), as well as religious delusions. The presence of violent content in the delusions, even if the violence was directed toward others, did not predict violence during the follow-up period. The duration of the delusions was not related to subsequent violence. None of the noncontent-related dimensions of the delusions was significantly related to violence at 20 weeks. Over the full year, however, the propensity to act on delusions in general (excluding violent actions) was the only significant association with a tendency to commit violent acts. No other MMDAS dimensions showed this relationship.

The presence of variables that might be expected to potentiate the impact of delusions on violence showed inconsistent effects on the rate of violent behavior. Thus, the presence of any hallucinations among subjects with delusions was associated with increased violence at 1 year ($\chi^2 = 5.52$, df = 1, p = .019), although the increase at 20 weeks was not significant. A similar pattern was seen for command hallucinations per se, with a trend toward increased violence at 20 weeks ($\chi^2 = 3.42$, df = 1, p = .064) and a significant finding at 1 year ($\chi^2 = 7.09$, df = 1, p = .008). There were, however, no significant interactions between delusions and scores on either the Schedule of Imagined Violence (see later) or the Hare Psychopathy Checklist—Screening Version (see earlier) and later violence. Despite analyses from this study showing a strong relationship overall between violence and substance abuse, delusional subjects who had diagnoses of substance abuse or dependence were not significantly more likely to be violent at 20 weeks ($\chi^2 = 1.49$, df = 1, p = .22) or 1 year ($\chi^2 = 0.08$, df = 1, p = 0.77) than were those without abuse or dependence. In contrast, among nondelusional subjects, significant increases in rates of violence at both points were found for substance abusers (20 weeks: $\chi^2 = 30.47$, df = 1, p < .001; 1 year: $\chi^2 = 32.62$, df = 1, p < .001).

The failure to confirm the predicted relationship between delusions and violence led to a more direct test of the TCO hypothesis. A subset of eight questions from the DIS screening questions for delusions were selected to represent the TCO construct. As can be seen in Part B of Table 4.3, contrary to what the prior TCO research would predict, subjects rated as having a TCO delusion were significantly *less likely* than were those without such a delusion to be violent both during the first 20 weeks and over the entire year after hospital discharge (20 weeks: $\chi^2 = 7.32$, df = 1, p = .007; entire year: $\chi^2 = 7.05$, df = 1, p = .008). (For a more complete explanation of the methods used here and for additional analyses, see Appelbaum, Robbins, & Monahan, 2000.)

Several methodological explanations were considered for the failure to confirm the results of earlier studies. First, the possibility was examined that the different criteria for TCO delusions used in this study affected the outcome. When close approximations to the criteria used by earlier research groups were constructed, however, highly significant correlations with our criteria were found, making it unlikely that these differences accounted for much of the variance. Second, we explored whether differences in measurement of violence might have accounted for the contrast between our findings and the earlier work. Previous studies had included less severe acts, not resulting in injury, in the category of "violence." Adding these other aggressive acts to our outcome measure, though, still yielded no significant relationship between TCO delusions and violence.

Two other methodological differences, however, may be of greater significance. The earlier studies all had examined the relationship between TCO symptoms and violence during some previous period. Our analyses focused on the prospective, predictive effect of the presence of TCO delusions. As with all retrospective methods, the earlier studies may have introduced unspecifiable biases into the data.

In addition, reported data from the earlier studies relied on subjects' answers to screening questions to rate them as delusional. Thus, for the most part, if subjects responded affirmatively to a question regarding, for example, whether someone was trying to do them harm, they were rated as having a TCO delusion. In contrast, the interviewers in this study were instructed to probe subjects' responses and to assess, on the basis of all data available to them (including the subjects' medical records at baseline), whether subjects actually were delusional. This process resulted in a reduction in the number of persons who could be rated at baseline as having TCO delusions from the 532 subjects who responded affirmatively to at least one TCO screening question to the 230 who were judged to have a TCO delusion. When we duplicated the approaches of the earlier studies by using retrospective analyses and relying on subjects' self-report of symptoms, we found that persons with self-reported TCO symptoms had higher rates of violence at baseline and at every follow-up interview.

Although with these techniques we were able essentially to replicate the results of the earlier studies, we could do so only by including a large number of presumptively nondelusional symptoms under the TCO rubric and by looking at the data retrospectively, with all the potential for bias that this method entails. Assuming that the relationship previously found between TCO symptoms (including both delusional and nondelusional symptoms) and violence is not entirely an artifact of the retrospective method, it is our belief that it may be accounted for by an association between a generally suspicious attitude toward others—with associated anger and impulsiveness—and violent behavior. Thus, when the effects of anger (using the Novaco Anger Scale [Novaco, 1994]) and impulsiveness (measured by the Barratt Impulsiveness Scale [Barratt, 1994]) are controlled, the significant association between self-reported TCO symptoms and violence is eliminated at every follow-up interview (Appelbaum, et al., 2000).

Conclusions Regarding Delusions and Violence

Contrary to popular wisdom and to the results of several other studies, the data from this study suggest that the presence of delusions does not predict higher rates of violence among recently discharged psychiatric patients. This conclusion remains accurate even when the type of delusions, their content (including violent content), and their noncontent-related dimensions are taken into account. In particular, the recent, much-discussed findings of a relationship between threat/control-override delusions and violence were not confirmed in this study. On the other hand, nondelusional suspiciousness— perhaps involving a tendency toward misperception of others' behavior as indicating hostile intent—does appear to be linked with subsequent violence and may account for the findings of previous studies (Arseneault et al., 2000).

These data, of course, should not be taken as evidence that delusions never cause violence. It is clear from clinical experience and from many other studies that they can and do. Our findings are however, probably in accord with those of Junginger, Parks-Levy, and McGuire (1998), who found in a survey of 54 delusional inpatients that "delusional motivation of violence is rare." This may be because, as Estroff, Zimmer, Lachicotte, and Benoit (1994) have suggested, delusions are often associated with chronic psychotic conditions, which are frequently attended by social withdrawal and the development of smaller social networks. Delusional subjects in the community, therefore, may have less desire and fewer opportunities to engage in the interpersonal interactions that can lead to violence compared with less severely ill patients. Although we cannot support this hypothesis with our data (controlling for social network size did not affect the relationship between TCO symptoms and violence), it is deserving of further exploration.

HALLUCINATIONS

The presumption of a link between hallucinations and violence is, if anything, even stronger than the supposition of a relationship between delusions and violence. Clinicians are taught uniformly during their training that patients experiencing command hallucinations, in particular voices commanding them to commit violent acts, are usually dangerous and in need of immediate hospitalization. As with delusions, there is no question that command hallucinations can result in violence (McNiel, 1994; McNiel, Eisner, & Binder, 2000), but it is less clear that people who hear such voices are at elevated risk of violence. Rudnick (1999), in a recent review, found seven controlled studies of the relationship between command hallucinations and violence, all of them retrospective, and none free of methodological problems. Interestingly, given popular beliefs on the matter, no study found a positive relationship between command hallucinations and violence, and one found an inverse relation. When violence did occur in the presence of command hallucinations, it appeared positively related to the benevolence and familiarity of the commanding voice and negatively related to the seriousness of the behavior commanded.

Measures of Hallucinations in the MacArthur Study

Hallucinations were ascertained in our study through a structured series of questions at baseline and at every follow-up interview. Subjects were asked whether they "more than once had the experience of hearing things or voices other people couldn't hear." If the subjects responded affirmatively, the nature of the hallucinations, their duration, their content, and the subjects' attitudes toward them were probed. Only subjects who experienced hallucinations in the last 2 months before admission (27% of the sample at baseline, n = 304) were included in these analyses.

What Was the Relation of Hallucinations to Violence?

In keeping with the existing literature, neither hallucinations in general nor command hallucinations at baseline (n = 164) were significantly associated with acts of violence during the first 20 weeks or over the full year of the study (Parts A and B of Table 4.4). Violence was also not associated with the duration of the hallucinations, the subject's feeling that the voices had to be obeyed, a history of having obeyed the voices, or the subject's belief that he or she would obey the voices in the future.

As shown in Part C of Table 4.4, however, when subjects reported that the voices actually commanded them to commit acts of violence against other people, they were significantly more likely to be violent in the first 20 weeks and over the entire year (20 weeks: $\chi^2 = 3.84$, df = 1, p = .05; entire

TABLE 4.4. Hallucinations Before Hospitalization and Postdischarge Violence

	% Violent	
Hallucinations	First 20 Weeks	1 Year
A. Any		
No	18.9 (n = 129)	27.4 (n = 189)
Yes	19.0 (n = 47)	29.0 (n = 73)
B. Command		
No	18.5 (n = 147)	27.1 (n = 219)
Yes	21.8 (n = 29)	32.3 (n = 43)
C. Command to be Violent		
No	16.6 (n = 32)*	23.9 (n = 47)***
Yes	27.7 (n = 18)	44.6 (n = 29)

* p <.05 *** p <.001.

year: $\chi^2 = 10.23$, df = 1, p = .001). This was true whether or not subjects had a history of having obeyed the voices commanding violence in the past.

Conclusions Regarding Hallucinations and Violence

Our findings regarding the connection between command hallucinations and violence are somewhat more in keeping with conventional wisdom than were the results on delusions and violence. Although command hallucinations per se did not elevate violence risk, if the voices commanded violent acts, the likelihood of their occurrence over the subsequent year was significantly increased. These results should reinforce the tendency toward caution that clinicians have always had when dealing with patients who report voices commanding them to be violent.

VIOLENT THOUGHTS

"Have you recently been having thoughts of harming other people?" For as long as anyone can recall, this has been a standard question of clinicians' mental status examinations for patients at admission and discharge from psychiatric facilities. Clinicians in training are taught routinely to make this inquiry. Indeed, failure to ask the question could be considered negligent if the patient harmed someone soon after the examination and the victim claimed that the injury could have been avoided with proper clinical inquiry about the patient's thoughts of harming others.

The logic for the question seems straightforward. For the psychodynamic clinician, the patient's affirmative answer provides evidence of aggressive impulses that may signal a greater risk of harm. For the cognitive–behavioral clinician, it suggests the possibility of scripts, that is, cognitive representations of aggressive patterns of behavior, that might be triggered by the patient's future social encounters.

Yet, for purposes of estimating the likelihood of future violence, surprisingly little is known about the actual value of patients' self-reports of their thoughts about harming others. Some research has examined the relationship between self-reports of thoughts of harming others and actual aggression among sexual psychopaths (e.g., Dean & Malamuth, 1997; Malamuth,

1998), as well as nonclinical samples such as school children (e.g., Rosen-feld, Huesmann, Eron, & Torney-Purta, 1982), adolescent delinquents (e.g., Silver, 1996), and college students (e.g., Greenwald & Harder, 1997; Kenrick & Sheets, 1993). The nature of these samples, however, does not allow one to apply their results confidently to individuals with mental illness.

Thus the predictive power of self-reports of violent thoughts by patients hospitalized for mental disorders continues to be a theoretical presumption. One of the objectives of the present project was to examine this presumption empirically by constructing and employing a method to assess patients' thoughts of violence and determine their relation to later violent acts. The results could provide clinicians with a tool for more systematic questioning of patients about violent thoughts, as well as a better grasp of the value and limits of their answers for violence risk estimates.

Measures of Violent Thoughts in the MacArthur Study

An instrument called the *Schedule of Imagined Violence* (SIV) was con-structed specifically for use in this research. The SIV is a structured set of eight questions with coded response categories (Grisso, Davis, Vesselinov, Appelbaum, & Monahan, 2000). Only participants who answered the first question positively ("Do you ever have daydreams or thoughts about physi-cally hurting or injuring some other persons?") were asked the remaining seven questions, which inquire about the nature of the respondent's injurious ideas. Each question inquires about a different quality of such images: Re-cency (question 2), Frequency (3), Chronicity (4), Similarity/Diversity in Type of Harm (5), Target Focused vs. Generalized (6), Change in Serious-ness of Harm (7), and Proximity to Target (8). Responses do not contribute to a total score; each question is examined separately.

Patients were assigned either of two categories, called SIV+ and SIV−, based on their answers to the first two SIV questions. SIV+ status required that they report ever having thoughts about physically harming others (Ques-tion 1) and that the last time this had happened was within the past 2 months (Question 2).

Patients received the SIV at hospital baseline and at each follow-up in-terview during the year following hospital discharge. SIV+ prevalence was examined for patients at hospital baseline by gender, age, ethnicity, diagnostic category, and symptom severity. We also examined the relation between patients' SIV status at hospital baseline and at various follow-up interviews in the community. In other words, what can clinicians safely infer about a patient's future violence after discharge based on their SIV responses during hospitalization?

Clinicians are aware that among patients who report thoughts of violence at the time of acute distress (that is, during hospitalization), those thoughts will continue for some patients after discharge while for other patients they will not. Theoretically this continuance or discontinuance of violent thoughts, perhaps even more than the presence of those thoughts during hospitalization, may be important to know for purposes of understanding patients' violent acts after discharge. Consequently, violence prevalence rates were calculated for two classes of patients: "SIV+ persistent," defined as SIV+ at hospital baseline and at both the first and second follow-up interviews; and "SIV+ Non-Persistent," defined as SIV+ at hospital baseline but at none of the five community follow-up interviews.

What Proportion of Patients Reported Violent Thoughts?

At baseline, 339 of the 1136 patients were SIV+. The proportions of patients who were SIV+ at baseline hospital interview and at each 10-week follow-up period in the community were 30% at baseline, 27% at 10 weeks, 28% at 20 weeks, 24% at 30 weeks, 22% at 40 weeks, and 21% at 50 weeks. Among patients for whom SIV data were available across all follow-up interviews, the percent reporting violent thoughts during at least one interview was 42% by 10 weeks, 49% through 20 weeks, 52% through 30 weeks, 55% through 40 weeks, and 57% through 50 weeks.

The proportion of SIV+ participants in various gender, ethnicity, age, diagnostic, and symptom severity categories remained fairly close to the SIV+ percent for the total patient group in terms of absolute percentages. Nevertheless, SIV+ prevalence among patients was significantly higher for nonwhites (94% of whom were African American and 16% of whom were Hispanic) than for whites (with socioeconomic status controlled), for younger than for older age groups, for patients with diagnoses involving substance abuse or dependence, and for patients with greater symptom severity (Grisso et al., 2000).

We examined the relation between SIV+ status at baseline and at various community follow-up points for the hospitalized patients. Several observations can be made about the results.

First, the percentage of patients who were SIV+ and who had been identified as SIV+ at baseline remained about the same (in the vicinity of 50%) at each of the five follow-up interviews. Second, at each 10 week follow-up interview, about one-half of persons who were SIV+ at that point had also been SIV+ at the previous follow-up interview 10 weeks earlier. Third, it is not surprising that at each follow-up point a decreasing percentage of patients identified as SIV+ had never been identified as SIV+ at some earlier point. Almost everyone who was identified as SIV+ during the year had been identified during the first one-half year after hospital discharge (i.e., about 80% by the third follow-up interviews). Fourth, about 20% of SIV+ patients were consistently SIV+ at baseline and throughout each subsequent community follow-up interview during the year after their discharge (Grisso et al., 2000).

What Was the Relation of Violent Thoughts to Later Violence?

The relations between SIV status at baseline and violent behavior during the first 20 weeks and during the year after discharge from hospital are shown in Table 4.5. The prevalence of violent behavior for the total hospitalized patient sample was 19% during the first 20 weeks, with a prevalence of violence for SIV+ patients of 26%, significantly higher than the 16% prevalence for SIV− patients. Similarly, the 1 year prevalence rate of violence for all patients was 27%, with a prevalence for SIV+ patients of 36%, significantly greater than the 24% prevalence for SIV− patients.

We found no significant interaction effects for SIV status by diagnosis or symptom severity. For both the 20 week and 1 year period, however, we found a significant interaction effect for SIV status by race and by gender. Examination of race by gender results indicated that the relationship between SIV status and violence derived primarily from nonwhite men and women, among whom those with SIV+ status were two to three times more likely than SIV− patients to have engaged in a violent act after returning to the community.

Finally, 41 patients were classifiable as "SIV+ Non-Persistent" (reported

TABLE 4.5. SIV Classification and the Frequency of Postdischarge Violence

	% Violent First 20 Weeks			% Violent 1 Year		
Variable	Total Sample	SIV+	SIV−	Total Sample	SIV+	SIV−
All Subjects (n = 939)	18.7	26.3	15.5***	27.5	36.5	23.7***
Race/gender						
White male (n = 360)	18.3	22.2	16.9	26.1	31.4	24.2
Nonwhite male (n = 178)	27.5	46.0	17.4***	37.2	57.8	25.9***
White female (n = 285)	12.3	10.5	13.0	21.3	21.1	21.5
Nonwhite female (n = 116)	22.4	35.0	14.7*	32.5	45.0	25.0*

* p <.01 *** p <.001.

SIV+ at hospital baseline but at no community follow-up interview), and 83 patients were classified as "SIV+ Persistent" (reported SIV+ at baseline and at follow-up interviews 1 and 2). Violent behaviors occurred during the first 20 weeks after discharge for 37.3% of the SIV+ Persistent patients, which was significantly greater than the 17.1% rate for SIV+ Non-Persistent patients.

Conclusions Regarding Violent Thoughts and Violence

According to our results, clinicians can expect about three in ten patients to report recent thoughts of violence toward others in examinations conducted soon after patients' hospitalization for mental disorders. Almost six in ten patients will, however, report violent thoughts sometime within a year (i.e., in hospital or in the year (after discharge). Clearly clinicians should not presume that patients who deny violent thoughts at hospitalization will be free of violent thoughts after discharge.

Among patients who report violent thoughts during hospitalization, about two or three in ten will report violent thoughts persistently during the year after discharge, while another one in ten will report no violent thoughts during that time. The remaining six or seven in ten were more variable in their reports of violent thoughts at various points after discharge. This suggests the need for clinicians to examine patients' violent thoughts periodically during community follow-up services to determine their persistence.

Our results indicate that when patients report violent thoughts during hospitalization, there is indeed a greater likelihood that they will engage in violent acts during the first 20 weeks and during the year following discharge. It was especially increased for patients who continued to report imagined violence after discharge and who experienced greater symptom severity in hospital. Clinicians should note, however, that the relationship is not strong; the difference between the prevalence of violent acts 20 weeks after discharge for in-hospital SIV+ patients (26%) and SIV− patients (16%) was significant but not substantial in an absolute sense. Moreover, the effects were found for nonwhite patients more than for white patients.

The results support the clinical use of patients' self-reports of violent thoughts as a factor related to future violence, as well as the potential value of the variable to improve risk estimates when it is used with other variables. They also underscore the need for further research to explain the relation of these findings to ethnicity, as well as the limits of this variable alone as a predictor of future violence.

Clinicians are encouraged to explore the use of the Schedule of Imagined Violence as a structured, systematic way to obtain information from patients about their violent thoughts. Most clinicians will want to know more than the answers to these questions in that the questions focus primarily on formal dimensions of violent thoughts (e.g., whether the violent thought is targeted or generalized) rather than on eliciting specific content of patients' individualized fantasies (e.g., specifically who they imagine they might harm). Thus clinicians would want to use the questions as an initial structure to guide further exploration of affirmative responses. Further research might examine the risk estimate value of certain specific items in the schedule (e.g., frequency, chronicity, escalation) that were not used in this study for SIV classification.

ANGER

Clinicians are well aware of the theoretical association between anger and aggression. From an empirical perspective, however, the nature of that relationship has been difficult to define. Novaco (1994) notes that the connection between anger and aggression is a two-way street, with each influencing the other. Yet the nature of that relationship is uncertain and potentially variable. For example, aggressive behavior can reduce anger (Konecni, 1975a, b) or, at least theoretically, can intensify anger. Anger does not always lead to aggression, and one can explain some aggressive acts without reference to anger. Any theoretical description of the relation between anger and aggression must recognize how they influence each other and why they do not always coexist.

To do this, Novaco (1994) has suggested that anger needs to be conceptualized into three psychological domains, which he calls the cognitive, arousal, and behavioral domains. These domains are not separate from each other, but rather multiple and interactive components of the concept of anger. Anger as physiological arousal—and its intensity and duration—is generally seen as related to aggression. Whether arousal is identified as anger, however, and whether aggressive action occurs, depends in part on the individual's cognitive appraisal and mediation in the process of perceiving the social circumstances that gave rise to the arousal.

There is no particular theoretical reason to expect that the relation between anger and future violent behavior would be different for persons with mental illnesses than for other persons. Past literature, however, offers little empirical examination of that "no difference" presumption.

Measures of Anger in the MacArthur Study

The Novaco Anger Scale (NAS) (Novaco, 1994) was developed specifically for use with persons with mental disorders. It is a paper-and-pencil instrument that asks examinees to indicate whether statements provided in the NAS are typical of their own thoughts, feelings, or behavior.

Part A of the NAS contains three clinically oriented scales that focus on cognitive, arousal, and behavioral domains conceptually related to anger. Within each of these scales are several subscales. In general, the Cognitive Scale contains subscales assessing focus of attention on potentially provocative cues, suspicion, rumination about provocative situations, and hostile attitude. Subscales in the Arousal domain focus on intensity and duration of anger, somatic tension, and irritability. Subscales in the Behavioral domain examine the tendency to respond impulsively, to be verbally aggressive, to retaliate physically, and to express anger toward substitute targets. Scores may be calculated for each subscale, for each of the three major scales, and for Part A overall. In the present study, we calculated scores for the three major scales and the Part A total score.

Part B of the NAS is based on an earlier instrument, the *Novaco Provocation Inventory*, which uses five subscales to provide "an index of anger intensity and generality across a range of potentially provocative situations" (Novaco, 1994, p. 34). These subscales examine primarily cognitive aspects of anger: perceived disrespect of oneself by others, perceived sense of unfairness, frustration, a tendency to see others as self-centered and insensitive, and sensitivity to incidental annoyances. Scores can be calculated for each subscale and for Part B overall. In the present study, only Part B total scores were calculated.

Novaco (1994) describes the extensive process that was used to develop the NAS, as well as its substantial internal reliability and test–retest reliability. Subscales within the NAS were substantially intercorrelated (0.35–0.55), but not to such an extent that they are redundant. Novaco (1994) reviews the evidence for the NAS' concurrent and prospective validity as a risk factor for violence. Although expected relationships between anger and violence were not substantial, they were significant and suggested that the NAS was a promising tool for testing hypotheses related to anger in persons with mental disorders.

What Patient Variables Were Related to Anger?

Table 4.6 shows the mean scores of patients at hospital baseline for the total sample and for various categories of gender, ethnicity, age, and diagnosis. Overall these means are slightly higher (by 1 to 2 points for subscales and by 4 to 5 points for total scales) than those provided by Novaco (1994) in his report of the development of the NAS with a sample of 158 California state hospital patients from three hospitals. Generalizing across scales, significantly higher scores were observed in the present sample for non-white than for white patients, for younger than for older patients, and for patients in the diagnostic group Major Mental Disorder and Substance Abuse than for patients in the diagnostic groups Major Mental Disorder and No Substance Abuse and Other Mental Disorder and Substance Abuse. Differences

TABLE 4.6. Mean NAS Scores by Demographic Groups

| Variables | Part A | | | | Part B |
	Cognitive	Arousal	Behavior	Total	
Total sample	31.9	32.8	30.2	95.0	69.4
Gender					
Male	32.1	32.3**	30.2	94.6	68.5**
Female	31.7	33.6	30.2	95.5	70.8
Ethnicity					
White	31.3***	32.5**	29.4***	93.3***	67.9***
Nonwhite	33.2	33.6	31.9	98.7	72.8
Age (years)					
18–24	32.5***	33.6***	31.6***	97.7***	70.1
25–29	32.3	33.5	30.8	96.6	70.5
30–34	31.8	32.8	29.8	94.6	66.4
35–40	31.6	31.7	28.8	94.7	68.3
Diagnosis					
MMD/NSA	31.0***	32.2***	28.8***	92.1***	68.0**
MMD/SA	32.8	33.7	31.1	97.7	71.2
OMD/SA	31.7	32.2	30.8	94.7	68.3

MMD/NSA = Major Mental Disorder and No Substance Abuse; MMD/SA = Major Mental Disorder with Substance Abuse; OMD/SA = Other Mental Disorder with Substance Abuse.

** $p < .01$ *** $p < .001$.

between the scores for men and women were less consistent across subscales, but, when differences were observed, women's scores were higher than men's.

Was Violence Related to Anger?

Table 4.7 shows the relation between NAS scores at hospital baseline and violent behavior within 20 weeks after hospital discharge and within 1 year after discharge. Subjects were divided into three groups on the basis of their Total Part A NAS scores: those below −.5 s.d. (standard deviation) for the total sample (Low; NAS score of 86 or lower), between − 0.5 and +0.5 s.d. (Medium; NAS Score of 87 to 103), and above +0.5 s.d. (High; NAS score of 104 or greater). In both the first 20 weeks and during the full year, subjects

TABLE 4.7. NAS Classification and Postdischarge Violence

	NAS (Part A)		
	Low	Medium	High
First 20 weeks	11.9	20.6	24.2***
1 year	17.5	28.0	38.5***

***p <.001.

with High Anger scores were twice as likely to have engaged in a violent behavior than were subjects with Low Anger scores, and this difference was statistically significant. No significant interaction effects were found for Anger category by race, gender, or diagnosis.

Conclusions Regarding Anger and Violence

The results provide limited new guidance for clinicians. We found that patients with high anger scores at hospitalization were twice as likely as those with low anger scores to engage in violent acts after discharge. The effect, although neither highly predictive nor large in absolute terms, was statistically significant. Clinicians, therefore, should use patients' anger, as they have always done, as a factor that incrementally increases their estimate of the risk of future violent behavior. The relationship was also sufficiently great to recommend the variable to researchers who seek multivariate indicators of risk of violence.

The Novaco Anger Scale, however, is not often administered in clinical settings. Moreover, it is not clear that there is a direct correspondence between patients' scores on this measure and signs of anger that are observable in clinicians' interviews with patients. Finally, we found that, among patients hospitalized for mental disorders, Novaco Anger Scale scores varied in relation to ethnicity, age, and diagnostic category. Some of these relationships (e.g., with age) are expected, while others (e.g., with ethnicity) are not easily understood and do not provide reliable suggestions for clinical use without further study.

CONCLUSIONS

In this chapter and the previous one, we highlighted findings regarding a number of "key" risk factors employed in the MacArthur Violence Risk Assessment Study. A few of the variables examined here were quite predictive of violence, as we expected them to be (e.g., prior violence). Other variables, contrary to expectations, were found not to be "risk factors" for violence in our sample (e.g., delusions, schizophrenia). Most criminological and clinical variables we examined, however, had a complex relationship to violence. Variables were associated with violence, but only among people of a given gender or race (e.g., violent thoughts, anger, living with the father as a child). For other variables, one component of the variable was associated with violence (e.g., factor 2 of the Hare Psychopathy Checklist; command hallucinations to be violent), while other components were not.

The complexity of the findings reported here underscores the difficulty of identifying *main effect* or *univariate* predictors of violence — variables that are across-the-board risk factors for violence in all populations. This complexity is no doubt one of the principal reasons why clinicians relying on a fixed set of individual risk factors have had such difficulty making accurate risk assessments. It suggests the need to take an *interactional* approach to violence risk assessment. In this approach, the same variable could be a positive risk factor for violence in one group, unrelated to violence in another group, and a protective factor against violence in a third group. Such an interactional strategy for violence risk assessment is the one adopted in the MacArthur Violence Risk Assessment Study and described in the next chapter.

5

CUSTOMIZING RISK ASSESSMENT

In the two previous chapters, we examined a wide range of risk factors for violent behavior in order to give the reader a broad sense of the personal, clinical, historical, and contextual variables that help to explain—or, in the case of delusions, fail to explain—the conditions under which violence in the community is more or less likely to occur. In emphasizing each risk factor one at a time, the chapters mirror the way in which research in this field often is conducted; that is, researchers tend to focus on a particular risk factor for violence without considering how each risk factor relates to others in influencing violence. Although this approach has led to increases in clinical knowledge regarding the effects of particular risk factors, it does not lend itself to the development of comprehensive actuarial prediction tools. Developing such tools requires that risk factors from multiple domains be combined in order to maximize predictive accuracy. None of the risk factors examined previously, taken alone, is remotely up to such a task.

In this chapter, we present an approach to actuarial violence risk assessment based on the use of classification trees (Gardner et al., 1996a). A classification tree analysis reflects an interactive and contingent model of violence, one that allows many different combinations of risk factors to classify a person as high or low risk. The particular questions to be asked in any clinical assessment grounded in this approach depend on the answers given to prior questions. Based on a sequence established by the classification tree, a first question is asked of all persons being assessed. Contingent on each person's answer to that question (or, depending on the nature of the question, on the answer found in each person's clinical records), one or another second question is posed, and so on, until each subject is classified into a high or low risk category. This contrasts with a regression approach in which a common set of questions is asked of everyone being assessed and every answer is weighted to produce a score that can be used for purposes of categorization.

In addition to its tree-based character, the approach we propose makes no pretense of classifying all persons into a high or a low violence risk group. Rather than relying on the standard single threshold for distinguishing among cases, our approach to risk assessment employs two thresholds—one for identifying high risk cases and one for identifying low risk cases. We assume that inevitably there will be cases that fall between these two thresholds, cases for which any prediction scheme is incapable of making an adequate assessment of high or low risk (Shah, 1978). Based on current knowledge, the aggregate degree of risk presented by these intermediate cases cannot be statistically distinguished from the base rate of the sample as a whole. By focusing actuarial attention on cases at the more extreme ends of the risk continuum, rather than across the entire continuum, our approach may increase predictive accuracy for the cases designated as extreme (Menzies, Webster, & Sepejak, 1985; McNiel et al., 1998).

In this chapter, we illustrate these ideas empirically. We begin by presenting a violence prediction tool developed using a standard main effects approach to show what the current leading analytic method produces in the full MacArthur data set. We then develop a tree–based violence risk assessment tool using a standard recursive partitioning software package. Next, we demonstrate how the idea of contingent risk assessment, when combined with a two-threshold approach to risk categorization, can be further operationalized to produce a tree-based actuarial model of violence risk assessment—the Iterative Classification Tree—that is more potent in identifying high and low risk cases than other approaches currently available. We conclude by applying these ideas to the development of a second, clinically feasible model of actuarial violence risk assessment. We do this by restricting the risk factors that enter the model to those commonly available in hospital records or capable of being routinely assessed in clinical practice.

METHODS

The sample size of 939 patients used in these analyses was obtained by selecting all subjects in the MacArthur Violence Risk Assessment Study who completed at least one of the first two follow-up interviews administered at 10 and at 20 weeks after hospital discharge (see Chapter 2 on the choice of a 20-week time period). The 134 risk factors that were measured during the target hospitalization are listed in Appendix B, along with their bivariate relationships to violence (as defined in Chapter 2, i.e., not including "other aggressive acts") expressed as odds ratios.

Statistical Procedures

Logistic regression was used to develop the main effects actuarial model. The dependent measure, violence during the first 20 weeks after hospital discharge, was coded as a dichotomous outcome. To derive an equation that maximized explanatory power using a minimum number of statistically significant risk factors, a forward stepwise variable selection criterion was used (a comparison of results using other variable selection methods—available from the authors—showed only trivial changes in predictive accuracy). The traditional $p < .05$ threshold was set for the selection of risk factors, and missing values were replaced by using mean substitution for continuous measures and mode substitution for categorical measures. The logistic regression equation was then used to compute predicted probabilities of violence for all 939 cases. Specifically, risk factor scores were weighted by the unstandardized logistic regression coefficients, summed, and then exponentiated to produce a predicted odds for each case. These predicted odds were then transformed to probability values using the formula $p = odds/(1 + odds)$.

To develop the classification tree model, we used CHAID (CHi-squared Automatic Interaction Detector) software available through SPSS (SPSS Inc., 1993). Specifically, the CHAID algorithm was used to assess the statistical significance of the bivariate association between each of the 134 risk factors and the same dichotomous outcome measure—violence in the community during the first 20 weeks after discharge—until the most statistically significant value of χ^2 was identified. Once a risk factor was selected, the sample was divided (or partitioned) according to the values of that risk factor. This selection procedure was then repeated for each of the sample partitions, thus further partitioning the sample. The result of the partitioning process was to identify subgroups of cases sharing risk factor attributes that also exhibited high levels of homogeneity with regard to the dichotomous outcome measure, violence.

To execute the CHAID algorithm, a number of decisions had to be made, including the setting of end-node splitting criteria, tree depth, and level of significance required for a partitioning variable to be selected (SPSS, Inc., 1993). In the analyses reported below, the partitioning process was terminated if a subgroup contained fewer than 100 cases, or, if more than 100 cases were present, the subgroup could not be partitioned into further subgroups consisting of 50 or more cases. In other words, no subgroup in the resulting classification tree was allowed to contain fewer than 50 cases. No limit was imposed on the tree depth, and the traditional $p < .05$ significance level was used as a necessary condition for variable selection, with missing values replaced using a method recommended by Breiman, Friedman, Olshen, and Stone (1984). The base rates of violence

TABLE 5.1. Main Effects Logistic Regression Model (n = 939)

Risk Factor	B	Odds Ratio
Psychopathy (0/1)	.876	2.40***
Child Abuse Seriousness	.427	1.53***
Frequency of Prior Arrests	.286	1.33***
Father's Drug Use	.779	2.18***
Threat/Control-Override Symptoms	−.412	0.66***
BPRS Hostility Rating	.127	1.14**
Prior Loss of Consciousness (0/1)	.551	1.73**
Employed Prior to Hospitalization (0/1)	−.530	0.59**
BPRS Activation Rating	−.164	0.85**
Novaco Anger Scale: Behavioral Rating	.038	1.04**
Involuntary Admission Status (0/1)	.500	1.65**
Violent Fantasies: Single Target Focus (0/1)	.628	1.87*
Grandiose Delusions (0/1)	.826	2.28*
BIS Non-Planning Subscale	−.031	0.97*
Mental Heath Profs. in Social Network	−1.704	0.18*
Drug Abuse Diagnosis (0/1)	.449	1.58*
Violent Fantasies: Escalating Seriousness (0/1)	.648	1.9*
BPRS Total Score	−.033	0.98*
Constant	−2.814	

BIS = Barratt Impulsiveness Scale; BPRS = Brief Psychiatric Rating Scale.
* = p <.05 ** = p <.01 *** = p <.001.

(i.e., percentage of violent cases) in each of the resulting sample partitions were used to derive the predicted probabilities of violence for all cases in that group.

To assess the predictive accuracy of the actuarial models produced by these methods and to facilitate further comparisons of our results with other research on violence risk assessment, we used a receiver operating characteristic (ROC) analysis. An ROC analysis consists of a plot of the sensitivity and 1− specificity pairs that are produced as a single decision threshold is moved from the lowest (i.e., all cases predicted violent) to the highest (i.e., no cases predicted violent) possible value. The ROC method of representing predictive accuracy is independent of the base rate of violence in the study sample (Rice & Harris, 1995b; Gardner et al., 1996a). The statistic used to summarize the ROC analysis is the area under the curve, which corresponds to the probability that a randomly selected violent patient will have been assessed by the iterative classification tree as being in a higher risk group than a randomly selected nonviolent patient (Swets, 1988; Swets, Dawes, & Monahan, 2000). The area under the curve varies from .5 (i.e., accuracy is not improved over chance) to 1.00 (i.e., perfect accuracy).

RESULTS

Table 5.1 displays the results of the logistic regression model. As shown, 18 risk factors were selected with the forward stepwise procedure, each of which contributed significantly ($p < .05$) to the prediction of patient violence. Table 5.2 presents a description of these risk factors and their bivariate correlations with violence.[1] Two of the risk factors listed in Table 5.1 appear to

---

[1] It is important to note that in Tables 5.1 and 5.2, no single risk factor can be isolated from the remaining ones as having an independent relationship with violence. For example, in Chapter 4, we report no bivariate relationship between delusions and violence. Yet grandiose delusions appears as the twelfth risk factor in the logistic regression model reported in Table 5.1. These results are not inconsistent. Only with 11 other variables maximally accounting for variation in violence does grandiose delusions come in to best account for the portion of the variation that is left. When all the variance is available, as in the bivariate test, there is no relationship.

TABLE 5.2. Risk Factors in the Main Effects Model

Risk Factor	Description	Pearson r with Violence
BIS Non-Planning Subscale	Barratt Impulsiveness Scale (BIS-II; Barratt, 1994)	.05
BPRS Activation Rating	Brief Psychiatric Rating Scale (BPRS) (Overall & Gorham, 1962)	−.08*
BPRS Hostility Rating		.08*
BPRS Total Score		−.04
Child Abuse Seriousness	Twelve self-report questions on the type of abuse a patient experienced as a child by his or her parents (0 = none; 1 = bare hand only, with no physical injury; 2 = with an object, with no physical injury; 3 = resulting in physical injury)	.14***
Employed Prior to Hospitalization	Self-report question regarding the patient's paid full-time or part-time employment status in the 2 months before hospital admission (0 = not employed, 1 = employed)	−.05
Father's Drug Use	Self-report question on whether the patient's father had ever used drugs excessively (1 = weekly/daily, 0 = less often)	.16***
Frequency of Prior Arrests	Patient's self-report of the number of arrests since age 15 years (0 = none, 1 = one, 2 = two, 3 = three or more)	.24***
Grandiose Delusions	Rating of the presence of grandiose delusions by trained clinical interviewers	−.01
Involuntary Admission Status	Legal status for the baseline hospitalization, as recorded in hospital admission records (0 = voluntary, 1 = involuntary)	.11**
Mental Health Professionals in Social Network	Proportion of social network members who were also mental health professionals (Estroff & Zimmer, 1994)	−.10**
Novaco Anger Scale: Behavioral Rating	Novaco Anger Scale (Novaco, 1994)	.16***
Prior Loss of Consciousness	Self-report of any loss of consciousness due to head injury on the Silver-Caton Head Injury Questionnaire (Silver & Caton, 1989)	.10**
Psychopathy	Hare Psychopathy Checklist: Screening Version (Hart, Hare, & Forth, 1994), a 12 item instrument, with each item rated by a trained interviewer on a 3 point scale (low = 0–12; high = 13–24). Following Hart, Cox, and Hare (1995b), subjects scoring 13 or higher on the 12 items of the Hare PCL-SV were catego-	.26***

(continued)

TABLE 5.2.—Continued

Risk Factor	Description	Pearson r with Violence
	rized as probable or definite psychopaths; all other subjects were categorized as nonpsychopaths	
Drug Abuse Diagnosis	Trained research clinicians using the DSM-III-R Checklist (1 = drug abuse diagnosis, 0 = no such diagnosis)	.17***
Threat/Control-Override Symptoms	Clinically validated affirmative answer to the following questions: (1) Have you believed people were spying on you? (2) Has there been a time when you believed people were following you? (3) Have you believed that you were being secretly tested or experimented on? (4) Have you believed that someone was plotting against you or trying to hurt you or poison you? (5) Did you feel that you were under the control of some person, power or force, so that your actions and thoughts were not your own? (6) Have you felt that strange thoughts or thoughts that were not your own were being put directly into your mind? (7) Have you felt that someone or something could take or steal your thoughts out of your mind? (8) Have you felt strange forces working on you, as if you were being hypnotized or magic was being performed on you, or you were being hit by x-rays or laser beams?	−.10**
Violent Fantasies: Escalating Seriousness	Self-report to the following questions: (1) Do you ever have daydreams or thoughts about physically hurting or injuring some other persons? and (2) Since the time you first started having these thoughts, have the injuries that you think about gotten more serious, less serious, or have they always been about the same? (1 = more serious, 0 = less serious or same)	.13***
Violent Fantasies: Single Target Focus	Self-reported answers to the following questions: (1) Do you ever have daydreams or have thoughts about physically hurting or injuring some other persons? (2) Are the thoughts usually about the same person, or might they be about many different people? (1 = same person, 0 = different)	.10**

* p < .05 ** p <.01 *** p <.001.

contradict findings from prior research. Specifically, Threat/Control-Override symptoms and the Non-Planning subscale of the Barratt Impulsiveness Scale were found to be negatively associated with subsequent violence. Both of these risk factors represent measures whose appearance in the literature on violence risk assessment is relatively recent. These findings suggest the need for additional research to further refine the role of these measures (see Chapter 4 on Threat/Control-Override symptoms). To assess the overall accuracy of this risk assessment equation, predicted probabilities were computed for each of the 939 cases, ranging from .002 to .93, with half the cases lying between .05 and .26. These probabilities were then submitted to an ROC analysis producing an area under the curve of .81 (p < .001; see Fig. 5.1).

Next, a classification tree model was produced (see Fig. 5.2A). As shown, the classification tree model contained 12 contingent risk factors that sorted the sample into 13 risk groups ranging in predicted probabilities from .00 to .59 (see Table 5.3 for a description of those risk factors not also appearing in Table 5.2). The ROC analysis, based on the predicted probabilities produced by this model, yielded an area under the ROC curve of .79 (p < .001; see Fig. 5.1). Thus, although these models arrive at assessment of violence risk using markedly different decision processes, they exhibit virtually identical levels of predictive accuracy (Gardner et al., 1996a).

We examined the effects of applying two cut-offs to each of the above models. For this statistical purpose, we chose cut-off scores with reference to the base rate of violence in the sample we studied. The prevalence rate of violence during the first 20 weeks after hospital discharge for the full sample was 18.7% (i.e., 18.7% of the patients committed at least one violent act during the first 20 weeks after hospital discharge). We defined any case assigned a predicted probability of violence that was greater than *twice* the base prevalence rate (> 37%) as in the "high risk" category, and any case whose predicted probability of violence was less than *half* the base prevalence rate (< 9%) as in the "low risk" category.[2]

---

[2] In practice, the choice of cut-offs (or "decision thresholds" [Swets et al., 2000]), for high and low risk must be made on substantive grounds by a decision maker legally empowered to do so. In Chapter 7, we present the decision maker with various cut-offs from which to choose.

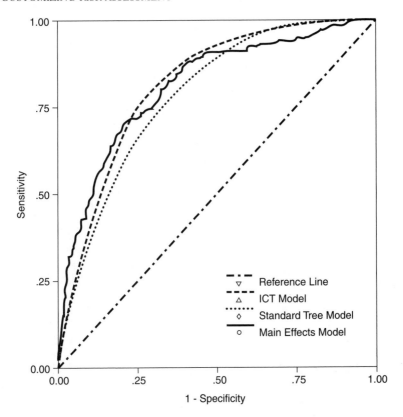

FIGURE 5.1. A comparison of receiver operating characteristic (ROC) curves: Main effects, standard classification tree, and iterative classification tree (ICT) models.

Parts A and B of Table 5.4 present the distribution of cases obtained by categorizing the predicted probabilities produced by the main effects and standard classification tree models, respectively, using the threshold criteria of twice and half the sample base rate to identify high and low risk cases. As shown, 42.9% of the cases (403 of 939) remained unclassified as high or low risk with the main effects approach compared with 49.2% for the standard classification tree model. In other words, use of either of these actuarial methods resulted in the classification of between 50% and 60% of the cases

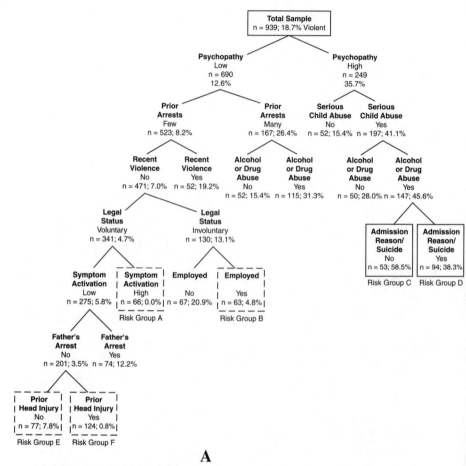

FIGURE 5.2. Standard classification tree (A) and iterative classification tree (A and B) models.

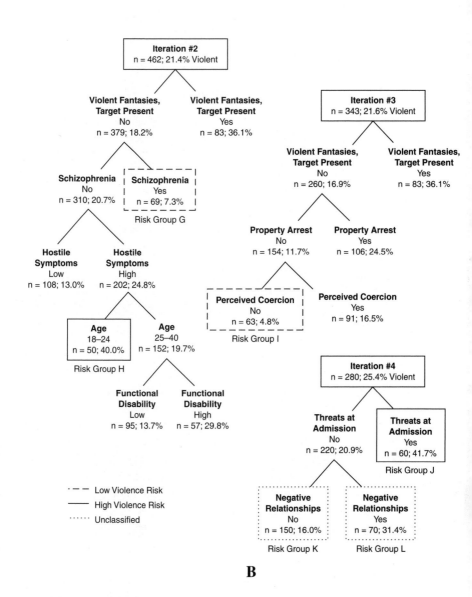

FIGURE 5.2. —Continued

TABLE 5.3. Risk Factors in the Standard Classification Tree that Are Not also in the Main Effects Model

Risk Factor	Description	Pearson r with Violence
Recent Violence	Self-report of violence in the 2 months before hospital admission	.14***
Alcohol or Drug Abuse	Presence of an alcohol or drug abuse diagnosis as measured by research clinicians using the DSM-III-R Checklist	.18***
Admission Reason: Suicide	Chart reviewing hospital admission records	−.01
Father Arrested	Self-report of whether the patient's father had ever been arrested or convicted of a crime (no = never; yes = at least once)	.15***
Prior Head Injury	Self-report of any head injury (with or without loss of consciousness) on the Silver-Caton Head Injury Questionnaire (Silver & Caton, 1989)	.06

*** p <.001.

as above the 0.37 threshold for identifying high risk cases or below the 0.09 threshold for identifying low risk cases.

Finally, we extended the ideas of a tree-based approach with a two-threshold framework to produce a tree-based actuarial violence risk assessment tool that yields a higher joint probability of classifying cases into high and low risk groups. Specifically, we reanalyzed those cases designated as "unclassified" using the standard classification tree method. That is, all subjects not classified into groups designated as either high or low risk in the standard classification tree model were pooled together and reanalyzed with the CHAID algorithm as described above. The process of pooling and reanalyzing cases was continued until no additional groups of subjects could be classified as either high or low risk. We refer to the resulting classification tree model as an *iterative classification tree* (ICT).

The ICT model (see parts A and B of Fig. 5.2) proceeded through four iterations (or reanalyses). After the first iteration—the point at which the standard tree model was terminated—the model classified 477 of the 939 subjects (50.8%) into either the high or low risk categories. After the second iteration, the ICT model classified as high or low risk an additional 119 of

TABLE 5.4. Use of Two Thresholds To Classify High and Low Risk Cases

| | Main Effects Model | | | |
	Low (<9%)	Unclassified	High (>37%)	Total
A. Observed				
Not violent	364	325	74	763
Violent	15	78	83	176
Total	379	403	157	939

| | Standard Classification Tree Model | | | |
	Low (<9%)	Unclassified	High (>37%)	Total
B. Observed				
Not violent	320	363	80	763
Violent	10	99	67	176
Total	330	462	147	939

| | Iterative Classification Tree Model | | | |
	Low (<9%)	Unclassified	High (>37%)	Total
C. Observed				
Not violent	444	174	145	763
Violent	18	46	112	176
Total	462	220	257	939

the 462 subjects (25.8%) who were designated as unclassified at the end of Iteration 1. After the third iteration, the model classified as low risk an additional 63 of the 343 subjects (18.4%) who were designated as unclassified at the end of Iteration 2. After the fourth iteration, the model classified as high or low risk an additional 60 of the 280 subjects (21.4%) who were designated as unclassified at the end of Iteration 3.

Iterating the original recursive partitioning solution, therefore, increased the number of subjects classified as high or low risk from 477 (50.8% of the sample) to 719 (76.6% of the sample) (Table 5.4). At the end of Iteration 4, no further groups could be classified as high or low risk; 220 subjects (23.4% of the total sample) remained unclassified as high or low risk by the model.

We refer to these cases as "average risk." The final ICT model contained a total of 20 contingent risk factors (two of which appear twice)—see Table 5.5 for a description of those risk factors in the ICT not also appearing in Tables 5.2 and 5.3—that formed 12 risk groups (6 low risk groups, accounting for 49.2% of the total sample; 4 high risk groups, accounting for 27.4% of the total sample, and 2 average risk groups, accounting for 23.4% of the total sample). Reanalysis of the unclassified cases thus resulted in identification of many additional groups of cases whose probability estimates for violence were above or below the thresholds of 0.37 and 0.09 set for identifying high and low risk cases, respectively.

Evaluation of the probability estimates for violence produced by the ICT model yielded an area under the ROC curve of 0.82 (p < .001), comparable with the areas under the curves obtained for the standard main effects and standard classification tree models (see Fig. 5.1). The ICT model was, however, able to classify 76.5% of the cases (719 of 939) as high or low risk. This compared with 57.1% and 50.8% for the main effects and standard classification tree models, respectively (see Table 5.6).

Of course, the iterative procedure described here is not specific to a classification tree approach. It also could be applied to the logisitic regression analysis described earlier. We performed such an analysis, extending the logistic regression in an iterative fashion to produce an iterative linear solution. Specifically, all cases not classified as above 0.37 or below 0.09—double and half the sample's base rate of violence—by the logistic regression equation were pooled together and reanalyzed in a second iteration of the logistic regression (the procedure ended at this point; see Steadman et al [2000] for a complete description of this iteration procedure). Iteration of the logistic regression procedure resulted in the classification of 62.3% of the subjects as high or low risk (up from 57.1% by the standard regression approach, but still far below the 76.6% achieved by iterating the classification tree).

Bootstrapping

We did not cross-validate the ICT model. Cross-validation requires that available data be divided into a "learning" sample (or model construction sample) and a "test" sample (or validation sample). Dividing the sample leaves fewer

TABLE 5.5. Risk Factors in the Iterative Classification Tree that Are Not also in the Standard Classification Tree or in the Main Effects Model

Risk Factor	Description	Pearson r with Violence
Violent Fantasies, Target Present	Self-report answers to the following questions: Do you ever have daydreams or thoughts about physically hurting or injuring some other persons? In the last 2 months, have you ever had these thoughts while actually being with or watching the person you imagine hurting?	.12***
Schizophrenia	Diagnosis of schizophrenia made by research clinicians using the DSM-III-R Checklist	−.12***
Age	Age at target admission	−.07*
Level of Functioning	Sum of self-reported ratings of the level of difficulty for the following activities: (1) housework by yourself; (2) stopping for food or buying things you usually need for yourself; (3) managing your money by yourself (such as keeping track of expenses, paying bills, or making money last until the end of the month); (4) using transportation; (5) making your own meals or cooking for yourself on a regular basis; (6) doing laundry by yourself. Response categories included 0 = none, 1 = some, 2 = a lot, 3 = unable to do it	−.01
Property Arrest	Arrests for property crimes since the age of 18 years as measured by official police records	.11***
Perceived Coercion	MacArthur Perceived Coercion Scale (Gardner et al., 1993)	.03
Threats at Admission	Presence of argumentativeness and threatening verbal statements at the time of admission to the hospital as measured by hospital admission records	.06
Negative Relationships	Average number of unique individuals named as involved in a negative relationship with the subject (Estroff & Zimmer, 1994)	.06

* p <.05 *** p <.001.

TABLE 5.6. Summary of Three Models

Model	Area Under ROC Curve	Percent Classified as High or Low Risk Using Two Decision Thresholds
Main effects	.81	57.1
Standard classification tree	.79	50.8
Iterative classification tree	.82	76.6

cases for the purpose of model construction, however, and thus "wastes information that ought to be used estimating the model" (Gardner et al., 1996a, p. 43). Thus, to estimate the extent of "shrinkage" likely to occur when the ICT model is used on a sample other than the one on which the model was constructed, we used *bootstrapping*.

Historically, there were two ways in which the stability of results was determined. In the first, the study was replicated, and the results from the replicated studies were compared with the original results. In the second, a theoretical computation of the variability of the results was computed by making assumptions regarding the distribution (i.e., normality) of the underlying data. Limitations exist with each of these methods. In the first, it may be expensive and time consuming to replicate longitudinal studies. In the second, theoretical calculations as yet do not exist for new methodologies, and the reliance on certain distribution properties may not be supported by the observed data. Efron (1979) and Mooney and Duval (1993) developed a series of computer-intensive statistical procedures, known as *bootstrapping*, to estimate the stability associated with analyzed data.

To understand how bootstrapping works, imagine that the MacArthur data set, with 939 subjects, was copied 1000 times. The resulting bootstrapped data set would now include 939,000 "subjects." From the bootstrapped data set, draw a sample at random of 939 individuals from the 939,000 lines of data. As the data are drawn at random, some individuals will be included more than once in this new data set of 939 subjects, and other individuals will not be included at all. The new data set has 939 cases, so it has as much statistical power as the original MacArthur data set, but has a different composition of cases. This new data set is analyzed, and the results of the analysis are stored. The process of drawing a sample of 939 subjects from the bootstrapped data set, analyzing the new data set, and storing the results is repeated a number of times. The variability in the stored results after the process is repeated many times (1000 in this example) can be examined to determine the stability of the original analysis.

This is, in fact, how we estimated the stability of our results. One thousand random samples equal in size to the original sample (n = 939) were drawn with replacement from the original sample. The ICT was then applied separately to each of these 1000 bootstrapped samples and the rates of violence in the risk groups observed. Table 5.7 presents the 95% bootstrapped confidence intervals for each of the 12 risk groups in the ICT model in order of decreasing risk. The ranges of these intervals indicate how the ICT is likely to perform on other similar samples.

TABLE 5.7. Bootstrapped 95% Confidence Intervals for the ICT Risk Groups with all 134 Risk Factors

Risk Group	% Violent in Risk Group	95% Confidence Interval	
		Lower	Higher
C	58.5	44.7	72.3
J	41.7	28.6	54.8
H	40.0	26.1	53.9
D	38.3	28.8	47.8
L	31.4	20.5	42.3
K	16.0	10.2	21.8
E	7.8	1.9	13.7
G	7.3	1.2	13.4
B	4.8	0.0	10.1
I	4.8	0.0	10.0
F	0.8	0.0	2.4
A	0.0	0.0	4.5

A CLINICALLY FEASIBLE ITERATIVE CLASSIFICATION TREE

Thus far, our presentation of the ICT method has focused on how well the method performed in making violence risk assessments under ideal conditions (i.e., with few constraints on the time or resources necessary to gather risk factors). For example, the risk factor that most clearly differentiated high risk from low risk groups was the Hare Psychopathy Checklist— Screening Version (Hare PCL:SV) (Hart, Cox, & Hare, 1995a). Given that the full Hare PCL-R requires several hours to administer—the Screening Version alone takes over 1 hour to administer[3]—and that it has to be administered by experienced clinicians whom Hare (1998) recommended should undergo 3 days of specialized training, resource constraints in many nonforensic clinical settings will preclude the use of what we will refer to as the "empirically optimal" ICT. In the remainder of this chapter, our goal is to increase the clinical utility of the ICT method by restricting the risk factors tested to those commonly available in hospital records or capable of being routinely assessed in clinical practice (see Elbogen, Mercado, Tomkins, & Scalora, in press). In other words, we attempt to create a "clinically feasible" ICT (see Monahan et al. [2000] for a full report of this effort).

The data analyzed above consisted of 134 risk factors. For the present analysis, we eliminated 28 risk factors that would be the most difficult to obtain in clinical practice, restricting ourselves to the remaining 106. Two criteria were used to eliminate risk factors. The first was to eliminate information generally unavailable to mental health personnel in the context of brief hospitalization (e.g., information in official arrest records as opposed to self-report of prior arrests). The second was to eliminate information that required the administration of a lengthy instrument, which we defined as an instrument with more than 12 items (e.g., a social network inventory [Estroff & Zimmer, 1994]). The risk factors that were eliminated in this clinically feasible analysis are indicated in Appendix B.)

---

[3] The Hare PCL:SV takes over 1 hour to administer as a free-standing instrument. In the context of a comprehensive clinical examination, in which many of the questions needed to score items on the instrument would already have been asked, the additional time needed to administer the Hare PCL:SV could be considerably less.

RESULTS

The clinically feasible ICT contained three iterations (Fig. 5.3). In the first iteration, the tree classified 429 of the 939 subjects (45.7%) into either the high or the low risk categories. In the second iteration, the tree classified as high or low risk 167 of the 510 subjects (32.7%) who were not classified into either high or low risk groups at the end of Iteration 1. In the third iteration, the tree classified as high or low risk 86 of the 343 subjects (25.1%) who were unclassified at the end of Iteration 2. At the end of Iteration 3, no further groups could be classified as high or low risk given the parameters of the model we had set (e.g., no group with fewer than 50 cases); 257 subjects (27.4% of the total sample) remained unclassified as high or low risk. The final ICT contained 15 contingent risk factors that formed 11 risk groups (4 Low risk groups, accounting for 50.9% of the total sample; 3 high risk groups, accounting for 21.7% of the total sample; and 4 average risk groups, accounting for 27.4% of the sample). Table 5.8 lists the risk factors in the clinically feasible ICT that were not already presented in previous tables.

The area under the ROC curve for the 11 risk groups in the clinically feasible ICT is .80 (p< .001). The distribution of cases that were violent or not violent during the follow-up as a function of the low and high risk cut-offs used to generate the clinically feasible ICT is presented in Table 5.9. Table 5.10 presents the 95% bootstrapped confidence intervals for each of the 11 risk groups in this ICT, in order of decreasing risk. The ranges of these intervals indicate how the clinically feasible ICT is likely to perform on other similar samples. The predictive accuracy of the clinically feasible ICT using a reduced set of 106 clinically feasible risk factors (an area under the ROC curve of .80) is comparable with the predictive accuracy reported above for risk assessment using the empirically optimal set of 134 risk factors (an area under the ROC curve of .82).

CONCLUSIONS

An illustration of the use of one of the ICTs generated in this chapter may be helpful. A clinician evaluating a patient's violence risk using the clinically

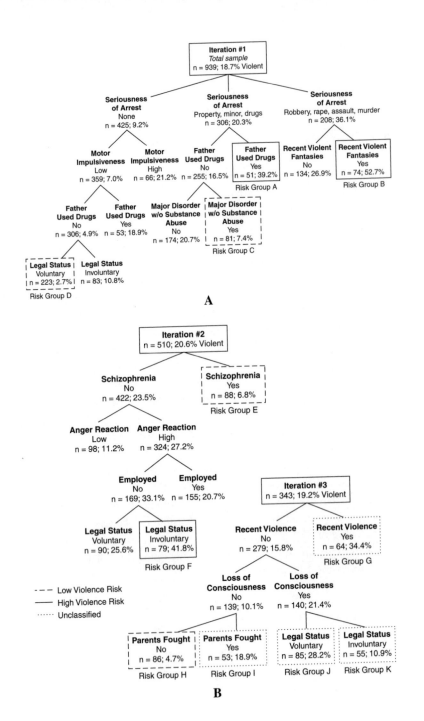

TABLE 5.8. Risk Factors in the Clinically Feasible ICT that Are Not also in One of the Previous Models

Risk Factor	Description	Pearson r with Violence
Seriousness of Prior Arrests	Patient's self-report of the seriousness of arrests since age 15 years (0 = none; 1 = minor offense; 2 = assault, robbery, rape; 3 = murder)	.25***
Impulsiveness: Motor Subscale	Barratt Impulsiveness Scale (BIS-II; Barratt, 1994)	.07*
Major Disorder Without Substance Abuse	Refers to a diagnosis of any major mental disorder without any co-occurring substance abuse diagnosis, as reached by research clinicians using the DSM-III-R Checklist	−.19***
Parents Fought	Self-report by the patient that his or her parents engaged in physical fights with one another when the patient was growing up	.06

* p < .05 *** p < .001.

feasible ICT presented in Figure 5.3 would first ask the patient about the seriousness of his or her prior arrests. If the patient stated that he or she had previously been arrested for a violent crime, the clinician would then inquire into whether the patient recently had been fantasizing about being violent. If the patient responded affirmatively to the second question, he or she would at that point be placed in the high violence risk category. More specifically, the patient would be placed in risk group B of Table 5.10, a group in which approximately 53% of the patients are expected to commit a violent act in the next several months.

If, on the other hand, the patient denied having violent fantasies, the clinician would then indicate whether the patient had a diagnosis of schizophrenia. If the patient did have such a diagnosis, he or she would at that point be placed in the low violence risk category. More specifically, the

FIGURE 5.3. Clinically useful standard classification tree (A) and iterative classification tree (A and B) models.

TABLE 5.9. Clinically Feasible ICT: Distribution of Violent and Not Violent Cases Using Two Thresholds

| | | Classification | | |
Observed	Low (<9%)	Average	High (>37%)	Total
Not violent	456	195	112	763
Violent	22	62	92	176
Total	478	257	204	939

patient would be placed in risk group E of Table 5.10, a group in which approximately 7% of the patients are expected to commit a violent act in the next several months. (See Chapter 4 regarding rates of violence being lower among patients with schizophrenia than among patients with other, often personality disorder, diagnoses.)

TABLE 5.10. Clinically Feasible ICT: Bootstrapped 95% Confidence Intervals for the ICT Risk Groups

| | % Violent in | 95% Confidence Interval | |
Risk Group	Risk Group	Lower	Higher
B	52.7	41.0	63.8
F	41.8	31.3	52.5
A	39.2	26.2	52.4
G	34.4	22.5	46.1
J	28.2	20.6	35.8
I	18.9	8.2	29.4
K	10.9	3.6	18.2
C	7.4	1.6	13.2
E	6.8	1.3	12.1
H	4.7	0.2	8.8
D	2.7	0.5	4.9

In this chapter, we have presented a new approach to the development of actuarial violence risk assessment tools based on the use of classification trees. Such an approach reflects an interactive and contingent model of violence, one that allows many different combinations of risk factors to classify a person as high or low risk (see Silver, Smith, & Banks, 2000).

We have demonstrated that this approach is predictively valid not only when applied to an empirically optimal set of information but also when applied to information that is feasible to collect in clinical practice. The predictive accuracy of the ICT using a reduced set of clinically feasible risk factors is remarkably similar to the predictive accuracy found using the complete empirically optimal set of risk factors.

Boosting predictive accuracy by combining models of violence risk assessment is the topic of the next chapter.

6

COMBINING CUSTOMIZED RISK ASSESSMENTS TO PRODUCE THE BEST ESTIMATE OF RISK

In the previous chapter, we described how a new methodological approach to actuarial violence risk assessment, the iterative classification tree (ICT), produced results superior in a number of ways to those generated by more traditional, main-effects regression methods. We illustrated the ICT method by generating two different risk assessment models from the data collected in the MacArthur Violence Risk Assessment Study—one model that was unrestricted in terms of eligible risk factors and one model that restricted eligible risk factors to those commonly available in hospital records or capable of being routinely assessed in clinical practice. Upon completing this work, we became concerned that the success of the ICT at assessing violence risk might be due to overfitting the data (i.e., capitalization in chance). This concern led us to estimate several different ICT models to obtain multiple risk assessments for each case. In this chapter, we show how multiple models can be combined to produce risk assessments that are much more accurate than any single risk assessment model taken alone.

What is particularly important in this chapter is not the specific variables in any given model. What is crucial is grasping the concept that by combining a large number of models, each of which contains a different combination of risk factors, the stability of the risk assessments for each individual is increased dramatically. That is, the final risk score for each case provides the clinician with greater confidence that the subject is in the "right" group. The other major point in this chapter is that by scoring each individual in many different models, more subjects can be categorized into groups with exceedingly high and low rates of violence. Although some of the statistical manipulations are complex, the basic conclusion is not. By giving each individual more chances to be either high or low risk, we are better able to classify them into groups whose extreme rates of violence are better suited for risk management decisions. This, after all, is the ultimate clinical goal of our endeavors.

COMPARABLE OVERALL ACCURACY, BUT DIFFERENT INDIVIDUAL PREDICTIONS

Although the two illustrative risk assessment models we generated in the previous chapter "looked" very different—that is, different risk factors entered into each model—they were remarkably similar in terms of their predictive accuracy: the empirically optimal ICT model yielded an area under the ROC curve of .82 compared with .80 for the clinically feasible ICT model.

Comparable levels of predictive accuracy, however, did not imply comparable predictions for individual cases. Table 6.1 shows the classification of individual cases into the high (>37%), average (between 9% and 37%), and low (<9%) risk categories by both the empirically optimal and the clinically feasible ICT models. As shown, of the 939 patients in the total sample, 352 (37.5% of the total) were twice classified as low risk, 109 patients (11.6% of

TABLE 6.1. Classification Based on Two ICT Models

	Clinically Feasible ICT Model							
	Low Risk		Average Risk		High Risk		Total	
Empirically Optimal ICT Model	No.	% Violent	No.	% Violent	No.	% Violent	No.	% Violent
Low risk	352	2.8	88	8.0	22	4.5	462	3.9
Average risk	72	6.9	75	26.7	73	28.8	220	20.9
High risk	54	13.0	94	37.2	109	64.2	257	43.6
Total	478	4.6	257	24.1	204	45.1	939	18.7

total) were twice classified as high risk, and 75 patients (8.0% of total) were twice classified as average risk. Thus, a total of 536 patients (57.1% of the total) received the same risk classification from both ICT models. In contrast, the numbers off the main diagonal of Table 6.1 represent cases whose risk classifications differed depending on which ICT model was used to make the classification. As shown, 54 patients (5.8% of the total) were classified as low risk by the empirically optimal model, but as high risk by the clinically feasible model, and 22 patients (2.3% of the total) were classified as low risk by the clinically feasible model, but as high risk by the empirically optimal model.

This observation — that different predictions may be obtained for the same individual from risk assessment models that have comparable levels of predictive accuracy — is not unique to tree-based models, but rather is a general property of actuarial prediction models (including main effects prediction models) (see McNiel, Lam, & Binder [in press] on prediction by multiple clinicians). Indeed, the only circumstance under which this observation would not hold would be when the predictions made by the risk assessment models are correlated 1.0. In this instance, however, the correlation between the predictions made by the empirically optimal ICT model and by the clinically feasible ICT model was only .52 (p <.001). The fact that these prediction models are comparably associated with the criterion measure, violence (as indicated by the ROC analysis), but only modestly associated with each other, suggested to us that each model taps into an important, but different, interactive process that relates to violence.

A TWO-MODEL APPROACH TO RISK ASSESSMENT

From this observation, a central set of questions emerged: What is the prevalence of violence among the cases *twice* classified as high risk, and what is the prevalence of violence among the cases *twice* classified as low risk? In other words, what is the violence risk for cases that both the empirically optimal ICT *and* the clinically feasible ICT classified as high risk, and what is the violence risk for cases that both the empirically optimal ICT *and* the clinically feasible ICT classified as low risk? Table 6.1 displays the rates of violence for each cell.

As shown, the Low–Low group had only a 2.8% rate of violence during the 20 week follow-up period and the High–High group had a 64.2% rate of violence during the same period. In contrast, the lowest and highest rates of violence we obtained with each of the ICT models separately were 3.9% and 45.1%, respectively. In addition, the area under the ROC curve for the two ICT models combined (0.83) indicated a higher degree of predictive accuracy than was obtained by either ICT model operating independently.

EXPANDING THE TWO-MODEL APPROACH: MULTIPLE MODELS

If combining two models predicts violence more accurately than either model by itself predicts violence, would combining more than two models predict violence still more accurately? In expanding a "two-model" approach to a "multiple-model" approach, the primary methodological challenge lies in how to combine the results of the various models. To explore how such combination may be achieved, we constructed ten ICT models, each of which featured a different risk factor as a starting point in building the tree (for a full description of this procedure, see Banks et al., in press).

Each of the 10 models was developed using the 106 clinically feasible risk factors (see Chapter 5). Model 1 was the same clinically feasible ICT model described in Chapter 5. The remaining nine ICT models were constructed with the same procedures as had been used to construct the clinically feasible ICT, with one exception: We forced a different initial variable into each of the nine trees.

More specifically, the procedure involved three steps. First, we had the CHAID program list "competitor" variables to the first variable that entered into the clinically feasible ICT (which was "seriousness of arrest," see Chapter 5). That is, we had the CHAID program identify those variables that would enter the ICT first if we eliminated "seriousness of arrest" as an eligible variable for the analysis. Second, from this list we chose nine competitors that were nonoverlapping in terms of the underlying construct being measured (i.e., we chose competitors that were not simply different indices of the same underlying variable, such as "alcohol use" and "alcohol diagnosis"). The variables chosen are listed in Table 6.2. Finally, we ran nine ICT analyses, each taking one of the selected variables as the initial risk factor to split the sample.

TABLE 6.2. Characteristics of the Multiple ICT Models

Model	First Variable	Iterations No.	Variables No.	Classified as High or Low Risk (%)	Area Under the ROC Curve
1	Seriousness of Arrest	3	12	72.6	0.803
2	Drug Abuse Diagnosis	2	9	65.6	0.738
3	Alcohol Abuse Diagnosis	2	13	60.7	0.764
4	Primary Diagnosis	2	8	55.3	0.753
5	Anger Reaction	2	11	62.8	0.778
6	Schedule of Imagined Violence	2	10	55.8	0.769
7	Child Abuse	5	14	56.0	0.791
8	Prior Violence	3	10	74.1	0.766
9	Age	2	16	53.2	0.784
10	Gender	2	14	62.7	0.806

RESULTS

Most of the ten ICT models required two iterations to complete, and the number of variables in each model ranged from 8 to 16 (see Table 6.2). Areas under the ROC curves for the ten models varied from 0.73 to 0.81, and the percentage classified as high or low risk varied from 55.3% to 72.6%. The specific risk factors included in each model and how often each risk factor was included are listed in Table 6.3.[1]

The next step in our effort to combine the results of multiple prediction models involved dividing the risk groups produced by each of the 10 models into 3 categories: low violence risk (<9%), average violence risk (between

[1] We eliminated one variable, race, from the final models on ethical and legal grounds. Race was included as an eligible variable in all ten models, but it emerged from the analysis in only three models: 2, 7, and 8 (Table 6.3). To avoid any possible misinterpretation of our risk assessment procedures as a form of "racial profiling," we removed the variable of race from the three models in which it emerged (with the next most statistically significant variable taking the place of race). The revised models without race differed only trivially in accuracy from the original ones that included race. For example, the area under the ROC curve for the original model 2, which included race, was .744, whereas the area under the ROC curve for the revised model, with race excluded, was .738.

TABLE 6.3. Variables Included in the Multiple ICT Models

Frequency Models	Variable	Model 1	2	3	4	5	6	7	8	9	10
10	Legal status	x	x	x	x	x	x	x	x	x	x
7	Major mental diagnosis and substance abuse	x	x	x	x	x	x	x	x		x
6	Prior arrests—frequency		x	x	x			x*	x	x	x
6	Child abuse—seriousness	x	x	x						x	
6	Diagnosis of schizophrenia, schizophreniform, schizoaffective	x	x		x			x	x	x	
6	Neurological screening—loss of consciousness	x					x	x	x		x
5	Age					x*				x*	
5	Anger reaction	x*					x			x	x
5	Prior arrests—seriousness	x	x	x			x			x	x
4	Employed full- or part-time	x	x						x		
4	Schedule of Imagined Violence (SIV)	x	x				x*		x		
4	Father's drug use	x	x	x		x	x			x	x
4	Lived with father until age 15 years		x			x		x			
3	Alcohol abuse diagnosis			x*				x		x	
3	Drug abuse diagnosis	x*	x*				x			x	
3	Gender	x	x		x	x	x				x*
3	Child abuse—frequency			x	x	x				x	
3	Diagnosis of antisocial personality disorder				x	x	x		x*	x	
2	Perceived coercion										x
2	Prior violence	x							x*		
2	Motor impulsiveness	x						x			

(continued)

		1	2	3	4	5	6
2	Parents fight with each other					x	
2	Valid attempt to kill self		x			x	
2	Sexual abuse before age 20 years		x				x
2	Marital status		x	x			
2	Threat/control override			x	x		
1	Prior hospitalization		x				x
1	Thoughts of harming self						x
1	Suicide threat present at admission	x					x
1	Father's arrests	x					
1	SIV—not frequent, not escalating, not while with target	x			x		
1	Age at first hospitalization	x					
1	Depression present at admission				x		
1	Years of education				x		
1	Hallucinations					x	
1	Functioning score					x	
1	Primary diagnosis	x*					
1	Decompensation present at admission		x	x			
1	Substance abuse present at admission		x	x			
1	Personal problems present at admission						x

*First variable in the model.

9% and 37%), and high violence risk (>37%) (see Chapter 5). We used the Ohlin/Burgess Scoring method (Ohlin, 1951; Burgess, 1982) to "score" an individual's performance on the models: Low risk was coded as −1, average risk was coded as 0, and high risk was coded as +1.

A composite risk score was then computed for each subject by summing across the ten models.[2] Each individual subject, therefore, had a composite risk score that could range from −10 (if the subject was in the low risk category in all ten models) to +10 (if the subject was in the high risk category in all ten models).

Actual composite risk scores ranged from −8 to 10, with a mean of 3.4, for the 176 individuals who were violent during the first 20 weeks after hospital discharge. Seventy-five percent of all violent individuals had a score of 1 or greater, indicating that across the ten models they were in the high risk category more often than they were in the low or average risk categories. For the 763 individuals who were not violent during the first 20 weeks after hospital discharge, composite risk scores ranged from −10 to 10, with a mean of −3.6. Although the composite risk scores covered the full range, 75% of all nonviolent individuals had a score of −1 or less, indicating that across the ten models they were in the low risk category more often than they were in the high risk category. Table 6.4 indicates the percent violent for each composite risk score, ranging from .00 to .90.

As two models predict violence better than one, so ten models predict violence better than two (i.e., the area under the ROC curve was .88 for ten models compared with .83 for two models). Are all ten models necessary, however, to achieve a high degree of predictive accuracy? To answer this question, a stepwise logistic regression was performed with violence during the first 20 weeks after discharge as the dependent measure. As shown in Table 6.5, only five of the ten models were selected into the stepwise logistic regression equation. The overall fit was very good (χ^2 = 300, df = 5), p <0.0001); c = .878; pseudo R^2 = .44). The coefficients in these five models are all essentially equal, suggesting that a simple summation of the scores

----

[2] Correlations among the risk categories emerging from the 10 models—that is, correlations among subjects' low (−1), average (0), or high (+1) risk scores in the ten models—were also computed. All models were moderately correlated with one another (from .26 to .57; all significant at p <0.001). Internal reliability (Cronbach's alpha) was also calculated and found to be .87.

TABLE 6.4. Violence by Combining Scores from Ten ICT Models

Score	No. of Cases	Violent (%)
−10	21	0.0
−9	52	0.0
−8	86	1.2
−7	9	3.8
−6	69	0.0
−5	72	1.4
−4	66	9.1
−3	71	12.7
−2	56	12.5
−1	40	12.5
0	47	21.3
1	54	22.2
2	43	34.9
3	41	43.9
4	29	34.5
5	20	50.0
6	30	66.7
7	23	73.9
8	20	70.0
9	10	90.0
10	10	90.0

TABLE 6.5. ICT Models Selected Using Stepwise Logistic Regression

Model	First Variable	B	Odds Ratio
1	Seriousness of Arrest	.638	1.89***
5	Anger Reaction	.638	1.70***
7	Child Abuse	.705	2.02***
9	Age	.679	1.97***
10	Gender	.693	2.00***
Constant		−1.4948	

*** = p < .001

provides predicted probabilities of violence very close to those produced by
the weighted coefficients of the logistic regression model. The alpha for these
five variables is .74.

When a composite risk score based on the five ICT models identified in
Table 6.5, is used, the 176 individuals who were violent during the first 20
weeks after discharge had a mean composite score of 1.9, and 50% of all
violent individuals had a score of 2 or greater. The 763 individuals who were
not violent during this period had a mean composite score of −1.8, and
50% of all nonviolent individuals had a score of −2 or less. Table 6.6 indicates the percent violent for each of these scores.

To increase the robustness of the multiple model risk classifications and
to produce the most parsimonious classifications possible, we used an analysis of variance to identify statistically significant differences in the percent
violent among the 11 different scores in Table 6.6, as well as a procedure
described by Nelson (1977) to yield a monotonic violence relationship.
These analyses resulted in the identification of five composite risk groups
(which we will call risk "classes" to avoid confusion with the specific risk
"groups" [or nodes] on an ICT and with the broad risk "categories" created
by our use of high and low risk cut-offs). The number of cases and percent
violent in each risk class are given in Table 6.7 and presented graphically
in Figure 6.1, along with bootstrapped 95% confidence intervals. The area

TABLE 6.6. Violence by Combining Scores in Five ICT Models

Score	No. of Cases	Violent (%)
−5	44	0.0
−4	147	0.7
−3	152	2.0
−2	142	9.2
−1	106	5.7
0	102	25.5
1	81	27.2
2	57	52.6
3	45	60.0
4	32	71.9
5	31	80.6

TABLE 6.7. Clustering in Five Risk Classes

Class	Score Range	No. of Cases	Violent %	95% CI (Bootstrap)	
				Lower	Higher
1	−3 or less	343	1.2	0.3	2.4
2	−1 or −2	248	7.7	4.7	11.1
3	0 or 1	183	26.2	19.5	32.4
4	2 or 3	102	55.9	46.2	65.3
5	4 or 5	63	76.2	65.4	86.2

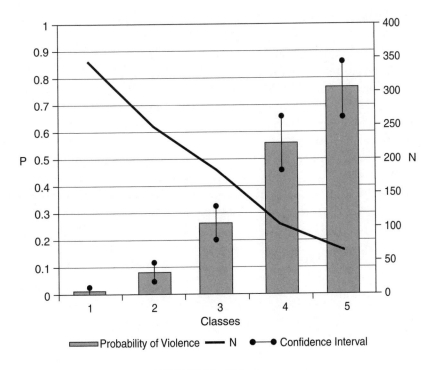

FIGURE 6.1. Risk classes.

under the ROC curve for the final five risk classes is 0.88, the same figure as obtained with ten models.

To further test the value of a multiple model approach to violence risk assessment, we asked two additional and related questions. First, is the multiple model approach as accurate in identifying people who were *repetitively violent* over the 20 week follow-up period as it is in identifying people who may have been violent only once? Second, what proportion of the total violence that occurred during the 20 week follow-up period was committed by people in the various risk classes?

In answer to the first question, it is clear that the multiple model approach discriminates among repetitively violent people in a significant and linear fashion. Overall, 6.9% of the subjects had two or more violent incidents during the first 20 weeks after discharge. From risk classes 1 through 5, respectively, the percentage of subjects with two or more violent acts was 0.0, 1.6, 9.7, 21.6, and 36.5 (p <.0001)

To answer the second question, we examined the 355 total violent acts committed by our 939 subjects over the course of the 20 week follow-up period. The results demonstrated that violence was strongly concentrated in the highest risk classes. Subjects in risk class 1 constituted 36.5% of the sample, but committed only 1.1% of the total violent acts. Likewise, subjects in risk class 2, while making up 26.4% of the sample, committed only 7.9% of the violence. The middle risk class, class 3, consisted of 19.5% of the sample and approximately the same proportion (23.7%) of the violent acts. Risk class 4, however, while constituting only 10.9% of the sample, committed 33.8% of the total violence, and risk class 5, in which only 6.7% of the sample were members, accounted for 33.5% of the total violence. The two highest risk classes taken together, therefore, contained about one-sixth of the subjects, and these subjects committed over two-thirds of the total number of violent acts committed by the subjects.

CONCLUSIONS

Rather than pitting different risk assessment models against one another and choosing the one model that appears "best," we have described an approach that integrates the predictions of many different risk assessment models, each of which may capture a different but important facet of the interactive relationship between the measured risk factors and violence. Using this "multiple model" approach, we ultimately combined the results of five prediction models generated by the Iterative Classification Tree methodology. By combining the predictions of several risk assessment models, the multiple model approach minimizes the problem of data overfitting that can result when a single "best" prediction model is used. As important, this combination of models produced results superior not only to those of any of its constituent models but also superior to any other actuarial violence risk assessment procedure reported in the literature to date. Using only risk factors commonly available in hospital records or capable of being routinely assessed in clinical practice, we were able to place all patients into one of five risk classes for which the prevalence of violence during the first 20 weeks following discharge into the community varied between 1% and 76%, with an area under the ROC curve of .88.

The multiple model approach to risk assessment appears to be highly accurate when compared with other approaches. It is also, however, much more computationally complex than other approaches. Five ICT prediction models need to be constructed, each with between two and five iterations and each involving between 11 and 16 variables (see Table 6.2). It would clearly be impossible for a clinician to commit the multiple models and their scoring to memory, and using a paper-and-pencil protocol would be unwieldy in the extreme, especially because many of the risk factors appear in more than one of the models. Fortunately, however, the administration and scoring of multiple ICT models lends itself to software. In clinical use, the multiple ICTs would consist simply of a series of questions that would flow one to the next on a computer screen—through the various iterations of each of the models as necessary—depending on the answer to each prior question, much as is the case in many common diagnostic tools such as DTREE (First, Williams, & Spitzer, 1998) and the Computer-Assisted SCID (First, Spitzer, Gibbon, & Williams, 1999). Under a grant from the National Institute of Mental Health, we are currently in the process of testing a prototype of such violence risk assessment software based on multiple ICTs.

The implications of the multiple model ICT approach we have described in this book for the clinical assessment and management of violence risk are explored in the next and final chapter.

7

VIOLENCE AND THE CLINICIAN:
ASSESSING AND MANAGING RISK

In the previous chapters of this book, we have described the goals, methods, and findings of the MacArthur Violence Risk Assessment Study. In this final chapter, we describe what we see as the implications of our findings for the clinical assessment and management of violence risk. We conclude with some general observations on the relationships between violence and mental disorder.

IMPLICATIONS OF OUR FINDINGS FOR VIOLENCE RISK ASSESSMENT

We were able, by using the multiple ICT actuarial methodology described in Chapter 6, to identify patient groups that differed, at the extreme, from having a 1% likelihood of violence to a 76% likelihood of violence in the first several months after hospital discharge. This finding far exceeds the most optimistic accounts of the predictive validity of clinical judgment (e.g., Mossman, 1994). Do we, then, recommend that the actuarial method described here be used *to supplant* clinical judgment of violence risk? Or, is the multiple ICT best considered a tool—a very powerful tool—*to support* the exercise of clinical judgment regarding violence risk? The question is not easily or unambiguously answered.

The group that developed another actuarial instrument for assessing violence risk—the Violence Risk Appraisal Guide (VRAG)—addressed the issue of whether, and to what extent, the results produced by such an instrument should be subject to "adjustment" by clinicians. Interestingly, their answer has evolved over time. In 1994, Webster, Harris, Rice, Cormier, and Quinsey stated:

> If adjustments are made conservatively and *only* when a clinician believes, on good evidence, that a factor is related to the likelihood of violent recidivism in an individual case, predictive accuracy may be improved. (p. xx, emphasis in original)

Four years later, however, Quinsey, Harris, Rice, and Cormier (1998) had a change of heart:

> What we are advising is not the addition of actuarial methods to existing practice, but rather the complete replacement of existing practice with actuarial methods. This is a different view than we expressed in Webster et al. (1994), where we advised the practice of adjusting actuarial estimates of risk by up to 10% when there were compelling circumstances to do so. . . . We no longer think this practice is justifiable. Actuarial methods are too good and clinical judgment too poor to risk contaminating the former with the latter. (p. 171)

Others in this field, while strongly approving of the use of actuarial instruments in violence risk assessment, have taken a more sanguine view of allowing clinicians to review and, if they believe necessary, to revise actuarial risk estimates. Hanson (1998), for example, has stated that "it would be imprudent for a clinical judge to automatically defer to an actuarial risk assessment" (p. 53), and Hart (1998b) has written that "Reliance—at least complete reliance—on actuarial decision making by professionals is unacceptable" (p. 126).

Two primary reasons are given in support of allowing clinicians the option to use their judgment to revise actuarial violence risk assessment estimates. The first reason can be termed *questionable validity generalization* and the second, *rare risk or protective factors*.

Questionable Validity Generalization

The VRAG was constructed and cross-validated on a sample that consisted entirely of male forensic patients, who were predominantly white Canadians.

The instrument has impressive validity in predicting violence among people with these attributes. Does that validity, however, generalize—at least, does it generalize as impressively—when the instrument is used to assess the violence risk of women, or of civil psychiatric patients, or of people of African ancestry, or of people (of either gender and whatever race and legal status) from the United States? This is a question of validity generalization (Cook & Campbell, 1979). Likewise, the iterative classification tree (ICT) generated by the MacArthur Violence Risk Assessment Study was constructed and bootstrapped on a sample that consisted of white, African-American, and Hispanic civilly hospitalized patients from the United States, who were between 18 and 40 years old. Is the considerable predictive validity of the ICT generalizable to people of Asian ancestry, or to forensic patients, or to people in Canada, or to people who are less than 18 or more than 40 years old, or to the emergency room assessments of persons who have not recently been hospitalized? The predictive validity of these two instruments may well generalize widely. Yet there comes a point at which the sample to which an actuarial instrument is being applied appears so fundamentally dissimilar to the sample on which it was constructed and originally validated (e.g., using the VRAG on the kinds of patients studied in the MacArthur research or using the ICT on the kinds of offenders studied in the VRAG research) that one would be hard pressed to castigate the evaluator who took the actuarial estimate as advisory rather than conclusive.

With regard to the ICT, we are confident in generalizing our results to American patient samples similar to those we studied. As the differences between the sample on which the ICT was developed and the sample to which it is applied increase, our confidence wanes. Generalizability is ultimately and obviously an empirical issue. Yet to say this is to beg the question of how far the instrument can be generalized now, before any additional research is conducted. One way to approach this question is to ask why, theoretically, one would think that the results reported here would *not* generalize to a given population or setting. For example, it is difficult to think of reasons why the ICT would not generalize to comparable patients who were in facilities in any location in the United States (i.e., not just in Pittsburgh, Kansas City, or Worcester) or why it would not generalize to people who were 17 or 41 years old. On the other hand, there are many reasons why the ICT may not generalize to forensic patients or to people with mental retardation or to young children or to the elderly. Caution rather than confidence would be appropriate in these circumstances.

A related question of validity generalization arises when one asks whether the results reported here can be generalized to patients with similar demographic and clinical characteristics in other countries, countries that may have very different (and almost always lower) base rates for violence than the United States. Although the *relative* level of risk assigned by the ICT may be similar in other countries, the *absolute* level of risk assessed by the ICT may be lower to the extent that the base rate for violence is less than the 18.7% in the first 20 weeks post discharge reported here. Here, too, caution rather than confidence is appropriate, at least until additional research has been conducted.

Rare Risk or Protective Factors

The second reason often given in defense of allowing a clinician the option to review and revise actuarial risk estimates is that the clinician may note the presence of rare risk or protective factors in a given case and that these factors—precisely because they are rare—will not have been properly taken into account in the construction of the actuarial instrument. This issue has been termed *broken leg countervailings* by Grove and Meehl (1996, following Meehl, 1954). The story is simple: A researcher has developed an actuarial instrument that predicts with great accuracy when people will go to the movies, and the instrument yields an estimate of .80 that a given individual, Professor Smith, will go to the movies tomorrow. The researcher then learns that Professor Smith has just broken his leg and is immobilized in a hip cast. "Obviously, it would be absurd to rely on the actuarial prediction in the face of this overwhelmingly prepotent fact" (p. 307). Although Grove and Meehl call the countervailing of actuarial risk estimates by rare events "one of the few intellectually interesting concerns of the antistatistical clinicians" (p. 307), they are skeptical about its applicability to areas such as violence risk assessment. In the broken leg story, they state, there is "an almost perfectly reliable ascertainment of a fact [a broken leg] and an almost perfect correlation between that fact and the kind of fact being predicted [going to the movies]. Neither one of these delightful conditions obtains in the usual kind of social science prediction of behavior from probabilistic inferences" (p. 308).

In the context of actuarial instruments for assessing violence risk, the most frequently mentioned "broken leg" is a direct threat, that is, an apparently serious statement of intention to do violence to a named victim. Assuming that most minimally rational people who do not want to be in a hospital can consciously suppress the verbalization of such intentions while they are being evaluated, direct threats are presumably rare and for that reason will not emerge as items on an actuarial instrument. Yet as Hart (1998b) states, "Does it matter at all what an offender's total score is on the VRAG, how many risk factors are present or whether he scores above a specific cut-off, if he also expresses genuine homicidal intent?" (p. 126). Similarly, Hanson (1998), in the context of predicting violence among sex offenders, has taken the position that "Although I am aware of no study that has examined the relationship between behavioral intentions and sexual offense recidivism, it would be foolish for an evaluator to dismiss an offender's stated intention to reoffend" (p. 61).

Grove and Meehl (1996) would no doubt respond that the "genuineness" of homicidal intent, or whether an offender has actually "stated" his or her intention to reoffend, cannot be determined with anything like the reliability of assessing whether a leg is broken, and, even if it could, the relationship between stated intention to be violent and violent behavior is much more tenuous than the relationship between being put in a body cast and going out to the movies (MacDonald, 1967).

In the context of the research reported here, consider the example of delusions. We found that the presence of delusions was not generally a risk factor for violence (Chapter 4), and delusions do not appear in the ICTs presented in Chapter 5. Yet we have elsewhere cautioned against ignoring delusions in a given case (Appelbaum et al., 2000):

> Even on their face, [these data] do not disprove the clinical wisdom that holds that persons who have acted violently in the past on the basis of their delusions may well do so again. Nor do they provide support for neglecting the potential threat of an acutely destabilized, delusional person in an emergency setting, in which the person's past history of violence and community supports are unknown (p. 571).

It may be instructive in thinking about this difficult issue, as it has been in thinking about other topics in this area (Monahan & Steadman, 1996), to analogize violence prediction to weather prediction. The National Weather Service (NWS) routinely collects data on "risk factors" (e.g., barometric pressure) known to be predictors of one or another type of weather. This information is analyzed by computer programs that yield what the NWS refers to as "objective" (what would here be called actuarial) predictions of various weather events. These predictions are given at regular intervals to meteorologists in local areas. The local meteorologists—who refer to the actuarial estimates as "guidance, not gospel"—then review and, if they believe necessary, revise them. For example, a local meteorologist might temper an objective prediction of "sunny and dry" for the forecast area if he or she looked out the window and saw threatening clouds approaching. A "subjective" (what would here be called clinical) prediction is then issued to the media.

Weather forecasting is one area in which the clinical review and revision of actuarial risk estimates has been empirically studied (for others, see Grove & Meehl, 1996; Garb, 1998; Quinsey et al., 1998). Clinical involvement actually increases, rather than decreases, predictive accuracy in the meteorological context. The clinically revised predictions of temperature and precipitation are consistently more valid than the unrevised actuarial ones (Carter & Polger, 1986).

Will clinical review and revision increase the validity of actuarial predictions of violence, as it increases the validity of actuarial predictions of the weather? Reasonable people will differ on the aptness of the weather analogy. As with validity generalization, above, the advisability of allowing clinicians to take into account rare risk or protective factors is ultimately an empirical question. A careful study of (1) *how often*, when they review actuarial risk estimates, clinicians feel it necessary to revise those estimates; (2) *why* clinicians feel it necessary to revise the actuarial estimates (e.g., the specific reason that the validity of the actuarial instrument is believed not to generalize, or the specific rare risk or protective factor that is believed to be present); and (3) *how much* clinicians want to revise actuarial risk estimates would be invaluable. Pending such research, we believe that actuarial instruments (including, among others, the multiple ICT presented here) are best viewed as "tools" for clinical assessment (cf. Grisso & Appelbaum, 1998)—tools that support, rather than replace, the exercise of clinical judgment. This reliance on clinical judgment—aided by an empirical understanding of risk factors for violence and their interactions — reflects, and in our view should reflect, the standard of care at this juncture in the field's development.

IMPLICATIONS OF OUR FINDINGS FOR RISK MANAGEMENT

We set out to study the assessment of violence risk in the MacArthur research, not the management of violence risk. The latter would have taken a very different design (e.g., a randomized clinical trial) than the one reported in previous chapters of this book. Yet it is a fair question to ask what a clinician is to *do* in response to a risk estimate generated by the multiple ICT method, even in response to a risk estimate that has been reviewed and potentially clinically revised.

At times, simply presenting and defending an estimate of violence risk may be all that is called for. For example, at a hearing to determine whether an individual passes the test of "dangerous to others" for the purpose of inpatient or outpatient civil commitment, all a judge may be interested in is the likelihood that the individual with mental disorder will be violent. Now, however, the principal use of violence risk assessments — at least in the civil context that we are concerned with here — is as an indicator of the need for violence *risk management*. In the not so distant past, a central form of managing a patient's risk of violence was to extend the length of the patient's hospitalization, often for months and sometimes for years. With the advent of managed behavioral health care, such a risk management option has all but vanished: Even patients estimated to be at high risk of violence to others may be discharged in a few weeks, or, increasingly, in a few days, assuming that they are ever hospitalized in the first place.

What implications do our findings have for the management of violence risk among those patients who may be briefly hospitalized but who will soon be discharged to the community? At the most basic level of risk management, our findings on violence risk would seem to have implications for determining which patients are most in need of *monitoring* in the community in the immediate postdischarge period (this would be called "surveillance" in public health terms).

In addition, our findings might indicate how one form of risk management—treatment to reduce violence risk—might be *prioritized* to make sure that those most in need of those services receive them. A prior question in this regard, however, and one rarely addressed (for a notable exception, see Swanson et al., 1997, 2000), is whether there is any reason to assume that receiving mental health services in the community is an effective risk management strategy.

Our data bear on this question. While we proceed with caution, given that we have not conducted a randomized clinical trial, we believe that our findings give rise to guarded optimism about treatment as one way to manage violence risk. We will briefly describe our ongoing analyses.

TREATMENT AND SUBSEQUENT VIOLENCE

We looked prospectively at whether the amount of treatment received during a given follow-up period affected the likelihood of violence being committed during the next follow-up period. *Treatment* was measured by a patient's answer to the question, "Do you receive any mental health or substance abuse treatment now [meaning as of this week]?" A patient who responded affirmatively was asked the nature of the treatment received and how many treatment sessions he or she had attended during the 10 week follow-up period.[1]

We examined the effect of receiving treatment during the first follow-up period on violence during the second follow-up period. Of the 752 patients who had access to the community during the first 10 weeks after discharge from the target hospitalization, 256 (34.0%) had attended no treatment sessions and 496 (66.0%) had attended at least one treatment session. For patients who attended at least one treatment session during follow-up period 1, the median number of sessions attended (including sessions mentioned in response to both of the treatment questions, above) was eight. For these analyses, we used classification and regression tree (CART) analysis (Breiman et al., 1984; Steinberg & Colla, 1995) to determine the point at which

[1] A patient was then asked, "Are you currently receiving any *other* mental health or substance abuse treatment right now?" As before, inquiries about the nature of the treatment and the number of sessions attended were made of those patients who responded affirmatively to this second treatment question.

to split the number of treatment sessions attended during follow-up period 1 to produce the largest effect on violence during follow-up period 2 (cf. Swanson et al., 2000). Using CART, we dichotomized the sample into one group that received six or fewer treatment sessions (including no treatment sessions) (n = 457; 60.8% of the sample) and another group that received seven or more treatment sessions (n = 295; 39.2% of the sample). The median number of sessions attended by the first group was 3 and by the second group was 12. The same contrast — attending six or fewer sessions versus attending seven or more sessions — was used to study the effects of treatment on subsequent violence for each of the remaining follow-ups periods.[2]

The relationship between treatment received during follow-up period 1 and at least one violent act being committed during follow-up period 2 is presented in the first row of Table 7.1. There it can be seen that of the patients who attended seven or more treatment sessions during follow-up period 1, 2.9% committed at least one violent act during follow-up period 2, whereas of the patients who received six or fewer treatment sessions, 12.0% — four times as many — committed at least one violent act (p < .0001). A similar pattern of results was obtained for the effect of treatment during one follow-up period on violence during the next follow-up period throughout the year after hospital discharge (see Table 7.1.).[3] The effect is statistically

[2] Medication only (without verbal therapy) was the treatment given to 1.4% of the patients in the group that attended seven or more sessions and to 15.6% of the patients in the group that attended six or fewer sessions. Verbal therapy only (without medication) was the treatment given to 35.3% of the patients in the group that attended seven or more sessions and to 29.3% of the patients in the group that attended six or fewer sessions. A combination of verbal therapy and medication was the treatment given to 63.4% of the patients in the group that attended seven or more sessions and to 55.1% of the patients in the group that attended six or fewer sessions. The difference in types of treatment given to the two groups of patients was statistically significant.

[3] In addition, for each follow-up period, the prevalence of violence was higher among patients who attended no treatment sessions in the previous follow-up period than among patients who attended one to six treatment sessions. For example, of the patients who attended no treatment sessions during follow-up period 1, 14.0% committed at least one violent act during follow-up period 2 compared with 9.5% of those who attended one to six sessions and 2.9% who attended seven or more sessions. For comparison purposes, Steadman et al. (1998) reported that the 10 week (i.e., one follow-up period) prevalence of violence among nonpatients living in the same neighborhoods as the discharged patients in Pittsburgh was 4.6%.

TABLE 7.1. The Relationship Between Treatment During Follow-Up N and Violence During Follow-Up N + 1

	Violent % (n)	
Follow-Up	No Treatment/6 or Fewer Visits	7 or More Visits
2	12.0 (47)	2.8 (8)***
3	8.5 (34)	3.5 (8)*
4	6.8 (28)	6.6 (14)
5	7.5 (33)	3.8 (7)

* p = .05 *** p = .001.

significant for follow-up period, 2 and 3, but not significant for follow-up period 4 and 5. Two more sophisticated tests of statistical significance — one employing propensity scores (Rubin, 1997) and one examining the effect of treatment in each of the individual risk groups described in Chapter 6 — confirm these findings.

Ordinarily, given the possibility of selection bias, there is much deserved skepticism when treatment effectiveness is inferred from nonrandomized designs. The propensity score analysis, which takes into account confounding variables that lead people to seek treatment, partially mitigates these concerns. It appears from these data that treatment in the community may significantly reduce the likelihood of subsequent patient violence and thus be one important risk management strategy. Do our findings give any indication, however, of which risk factors might be the most appropriate targets of clinical intervention to manage violence risk (Binder & McNiel, 1999; Heilbrun & Peters, 2000; Hoyer, 2000)?

Many recent approaches integrate risk assessment and risk reduction (i.e., treatment), usually by focusing on dynamic or changeable risk factors during the assessment phase and then by modifying those dynamic or changeable risk factors during the treatment phase (e.g., Webster, Douglas, Belfrage, & Link, 2000). We have taken a different tack. Rather than integrate risk assessment and treatment, we differentiate them. As Kraemer et al. (1997) point out, the process of assessing risk is fundamentally different from the process of reducing it. The former involves attending to all risk factors. The latter requires attending not to all risk factors, but only to those risk factors that (1) are changeable and that (2) when changed result in a change in the criterion—lowered violence risk. Kraemer et al. refer to these as "causal risk factors" and state that "structuring effective treatment requires a focus on causal risk factors" (1997, p. 343; see Carson, 1977; Heilbrun, 1997). In this research, we pursued the most accurate risk assessment possible, using whatever risk factors—fixed or changeable—best accomplished this task. We viewed the reduction of the violence risk that we identified as a crucial issue, but one best addressed on its own merits, separate from the issue of risk assessment.

Although our research was clearly focused on who to assign risk management resources rather than on how those resources should be deployed, some substantive implications for treatment as a form of risk management may be found in our data. One could ask which of the risk factors that we have identified are changeable and which, when changed, can be expected—based on other research (e.g., Roth, 1985; Bloom, Mueser, & Müller-Isberner, 2000; Crowner, 2000; Gunn, 2000)—to lead to a reduction in violence risk. Given the tree-based strategy we have adopted here, however, different patients may arrive at the same risk category by the application of very different risk factors. Indeed, we have not only relied on a tree-based strategy in our analyses, we have iterated the trees and then analyzed each case across multiple iterated trees. Therefore, trying to identify—even speculatively—which risk factors are "causal" from among the large number of contingent risk factors that are applied to any given case is not a productive strategy.

"Clues" (Monahan & Appelbaum, 2000) as to possible risk factors with treatment implications may still, however, be found in the MacArthur data. One way to do this is by examining the bivariate relationships between individual risk factors and violence reported in Appendix B. A second source of clues to treatment-relevant risk factors is the logistic regression reported in Table 5.1. For example, in both Appendix B and in Table 5.1, substance abuse, anger, and violent fantasies stand out as candidates for being targets of violence risk reduction efforts. Further research into the violence-reduction potential of treatments for co-occurring mental and substance abuse disorders (along the promising lines of Drake, Mercer-McFadden, Mueser, McHugo, & Bond, 1998) and for anger control problems (along the promising lines of Novaco, 1997) seems clearly indicated. Research on violent fantasies is only now beginning (Grisso et al., 2000).

A third way to identify possible targets for treatment interventions to manage violence risk is to consider the risk factors that distinguish the five risk groups generated by the multiple ICT in Chapter 6. A stepwise multiple regression analysis, into which all 134 risk factors described in Chapter 5 were entered, was performed to predict membership in one of the five risk groups. The results are presented in Table 7.2 ($R^2 = .613$). There it can be seen that while many of the risk factors are fixed (e.g., father's drug use and arrest history), others are potentially treatable and that treatment might have pay-off for violence risk management. Some of the risk factors that appear in Table 7.2 a clinician would not desire to change in the indicated direc-

TABLE 7.2. Stepwise Regression Predicting Membership in the Five Multiple ICT Risk Groups

Risk Factors	Beta
Fixed	
Frequency of prior arrests	.360***
Father's drug use	.523***
Legal status	.518***
Loss of consciousness	.266***
Abused as a child	.160***
Father arrested	.116**
Age	−.015**
Violence at admission	.223*
Treatable	
Anger—behavioral domain	.037***
Research diagnosis of schizophrenia	−.586***
Research diagnosis of drug abuse	.317***
Employed	−.274***
Research diagnosis of alcohol abuse	.268***
Violent fantasies	.187**
Suicide attempt	−.190*

* $p = .05$ ** $p = .01$ *** $p = .001$.

tion. For example, people with a diagnosis of schizophrenia or who are suicidal are less likely to be in one of the higher violence risk groups. No one would want to promote these conditions as a technique for managing violence risk. Other risk factors, however, have practical implications for treatment. Once again—and for the third time—substance abuse, anger, and violent fantasies emerge as predictors of violence risk. In addition, being unemployed and reporting having been physically abused as a child predict violence risk. Intervention programs supporting employment for people with mental disorder are reviewed in Bonnie and Monahan (1997). While having been abused as a child is a historical fact that cannot be changed, the abuse may still bear an important indirect relationship to violence risk, because, for example, sequelae of the abuse may include fear, anger, and inability to establish trusting relationships—all of which alone or in interaction may potentiate violent behavior. These sequelae of trauma may be changeable and may respond to treatment (Monahan & Appelbaum, 2000).

We emphasize, again, that our research was designed for the purpose of improving violence risk assessment. It did not extend to clinical trials attempting to change any risk factor we identified, or, furthermore, to studies attempting to test whether a change in a risk factor resulted in a corresponding change in the subsequent likelihood of violence. Definitive answers to questions about the treatment of violence will have to await studies with experimental or quasiexperimental research designs. Heuristic analyses such as the ones we present here, however, may be valuable in suggesting which risk factors might most profitably be the targets of clinical risk-reduction research.

CONCLUSIONS

The findings of this study underscore some important aspects of the nature of violence among persons with mental illness—and, in all likelihood, among other people as well. These relate to the causes of violence, our ability to predict its occurrence, and the interventions that are likely to lead to its control.

A historical view of the study of violence by persons with mental illness reveals a determined quest for the single variable (or sometimes a small set of variables) that will determine whether a person will act aggressively toward others. Once in hand, knowledge of this variable would lead inexorably to strategies for prediction or control. Among the causative factors postulated at one point or another have been electrical discharges in the temporal lobe; physical abuse in childhood; a vulnerability to shame; overcontrol of violent impulses or its opposite, the failure to inhibit their expression; and, most recently, for the people with mental illness in particular, the presence of one or another set of psychotic symptoms.

In its similarity to Koch's search for the single bacterium that causes tuberculosis and Ehrlich's pursuit of the "magic bullet" that would target the spirochete that gives rise to syphilis, this strategy evidences a desire to transfer to the study of human behavior the strategies that proved so successful in the early years of medical science. Perhaps unsurprisingly, the complexity of human behavior has thus far frustrated these attempts to find unitary causes of and solutions to violence. The data presented in this volume confirm that this pursuit of single causes of violence should long since have been abandoned.

Of the scores of variables whose relationship with violence we studied in this project, many (indeed most) had some significant association with future violence. None of these relationships was sufficiently strong, however, for it to be fairly said that a given variable constituted *the* cause of violence, even for a subgroup of patients. Nor, as the iterated tree models we used clearly demonstrate, does any single concatenation of variables account for violence as a unitary phenomenon. Our data are most consistent with the view that the propensity for violence is the result of the accumulation of risk factors, no one of which is either necessary or sufficient for a person to behave aggressively toward others. People will be violent by virtue of the presence of different sets of risk factors. There is no single path in a person's life that leads to an act of violence.

This conclusion has clear implications for future research on violence, as well as for efforts to predict and to prevent violent behavior. Research targeting one or a small number of variables, as so many studies have in the past, is unlikely to yield much clarity regarding causal influences or predictive strategies. Advances in understanding or predictive accuracy are more likely to come from efforts to assess the interactions among substantial numbers of variables associated with violence. Such studies often will involve large samples and complex assessment and measurement techniques. They usually will be lengthy and expensive and interdisciplinary.

Prediction is similarly fraught. It is no longer reasonable to expect clinicians unaided to be able to identify the variables that may be influential for a particular person, integrate that information, and arrive at a valid estimate of the person's risk for violence. If multivariate models hold the only hope of improving predictive accuracy—and our analysis of iterative classification trees suggests that, even so, no single model is sufficient, but the concurrent use of multiple models holds great promise—clinicians will need to have computer support available. At best, predictions will involve approximations of the degree of risk presented by a person, presented as a range rather than a single number, with the recognition that not every person thus classified, even one accurately determined to be in a high risk group, will commit a violent act.

As a necessary consequence of all this, no single intervention is likely to enable the successful management of potential violence. Multiple targets for intervention will exist, and they will differ from person to person. The multivariate interactive causal model of violence that is most consistent with our data also, however, implies that effective interventions need not eliminate all or even most of a person's risk factors. It should be sufficient only to reduce the presence or effect of these factors below the threshold (admittedly indeterminate at this point) at which their combined effect is likely to cross the threshold at which violence occurs. Although clearly it will be necessary to identify mutable characteristics of violence risk at which to target these interventions, not all need be effectively addressed for violence prevention to succeed. This should be taken as a bit of optimism in what to date has been an area bereft of much encouragement.

In sum, we believe that this study not only permits us to say something meaningful about techniques for improving the prediction of violence today but also suggests how we might best think about the problem of violence in the future.

APPENDIX A

This appendix presents the design and procedures of the MacArthur Violence Risk Assessment Study, providing details about instrumentation and data collection that will enable the interested reader to better interpret the findings presented.

METHODOLOGY OVERVIEW

Project Structure

The project structure had lead researchers at each data collection site who provided on-site oversight of the project, arranged access for data collection, and hired the field staff. Field staff included a site coordinator, research interviewers, one clinically trained interviewer, and support staff. The site coordinator supervised all on-site enrollment and data collection performed by the research interviewers (three to eight persons at a given time per site) and the clinically trained interviewer, along with maintaining consistency in the collection and handling of the data. A consultant psychiatrist was retained to review any differences between the diagnosis of the clinically trained interviewer and the chart diagnoses.

Efforts at the research sites were coordinated by a core staff at Policy Research Associates, Inc. (PRA) in Delmar, New York. PRA provided the central link for the sites and included a project coordinator who met regularly with the site coordinators as a group to discuss instruments, coding, and procedure decisions, as well as on-site feedback on instrument administration for all interviewers. Central staff were also responsible for cleaning and reviewing all completed instruments before data entry as a final quality control measure. All data management and analyses were conducted at PRA. Considerable emphasis was placed on the coordination effort and communication among all sites. Regular, project-wide meetings were held, and much time and effort were devoted to interviewer training and reliability studies. Reliability studies involved videotaped interviews that were circulated and coded in a systematic fashion among all the interviewers.

Pilot Study

After considerable instrument development, questions arose regarding the feasibility of conducting a very large study of risk factors for violence. How would patients react to the lengthy instrument that had been developed? How often should we interview discharged patients in the community? How much violence could we expect to find with the measures we had developed, and, given the prevalence rate observed, how large a sample size would be required for the analysis? Many of these questions were answered by a pilot study (for a fuller description of the pilot study, see Steadman et al., 1994).

The pilot study involved the investigation of risk factors that had been associated with violence in prior research, were believed to be associated with violence by experienced clinicians, or were hypothesized to be related to violence by contemporary theories. When a reliable measure for a key risk factor did not already exist, the MacArthur Research Network on Mental Health and the Law commissioned an expert in the field to develop a measure that would be appropriate for use with a population of people with mental disorder. Specifically, instrument development was commissioned in the area of anger (Raymond Novaco), psychopathy (Robert Hare), delusions (Pamela Taylor), and social support (Sue Estroff). Results from these instrument development studies, and reviews of existing measures of other risk factors, were published in an earlier volume (Monahan & Steadman, 1994).

The pilot study was undertaken at three sites (Kansas City, MO; Pittsburgh, PA; and Worcester, MA).[1] We selected a group of 169 patients admitted to acute civil psychiatric hospitals and administered a baseline interview in the hospital and re-interviewed the patients at regular intervals after discharge to the community.

We found that we were able to interview subjects in the hospital with our lengthy protocol and were able to locate subjects in the community for the follow-up interviews with acceptable rates of attrition. The level of violence observed during the pilot study led us to include female patients in the final design, as women's rate of violence was comparable with that of men, and to exclude patients over 40 years old, as the rate of violence among this group was substantially lower than that among younger patients.

The pilot test of our methods and procedures proved useful as well. We varied the length of follow-up periods—ranging from twice per month to once in 3 months—trying to optimize the period between our contacts with the patients in the community. We concluded that between 2 and 3 months was the optimum time between interviews. A longer period risked compromising patients' ability to recall events, and a shorter period was not cost effective. Collateral interviews were introduced to check the reliability of the data collected from the patients and to determine whether enough additional information was gained from the collaterals to include them in the final study design. We concluded that collaterals provided a sufficient amount of otherwise unavailable information to justify their retention.

Final Design

Based on the pilot study, we decided that approximately 1000 male and female acute civil patients between 18 and 40 years old would be enrolled

[1] Initially, we planned to study violence risk assessment among both civil patients and mentally disordered offenders. In a pilot study at two sites, in Maryland and Florida, we selected a group of insanity acquittees who were about to be released to the community and followed the same procedures regarding the baseline and follow-up interviews described above. The instruments developed primarily for the civil patients were, however, problematic when applied to the criminal patients. The fact that the insanity acquittees had been institutionalized for often very lengthy stays made many of the historical questions inapplicable. The high level at which the criminal patients were monitored in the community made their assessment very different from that of the civil patients. We ultimately determined that our design and instrumentation would need to be substantially modified to adapt to the criminal patients, and we chose to limit our study to civil patients.

at three sites, chosen for their geographic and patient diversity. This number would allow the statistical power necessary to perform the planned analyses. The patients would receive a baseline interview in the hospital and subsequent interviews every 10 weeks during their first year after discharge. Interviews would include assessment of a wide variety of risk factors as well as the violence outcome measure (described fully in Chapter 2). Patient self-reports would be augmented by reports from collaterals and by police and hospital records.[2]

Instruments

The risk factors included in the final design can be categorized into four general domains: personal or dispositional factors (e.g., age, gender, and head injury); historical or developmental factors (e.g., family, work, mental hospitalization, and violence history); contextual or situational factors (e.g., social supports, social networks, and stress); and clinical or symptom factors (e.g., diagnoses, functioning, and substance use). The risk factors measured in the MacArthur Violence Risk Assessment Study are listed in detail in Appendix B.

The criterion measure was physical violence to others by the discharged patient in the community. Multiple measures were used to create a comprehensive reconciled version of the violence that occurred during each 10 week follow-up period postdischarge. This measure is discussed in Chapter 2.

Training and Reliability

Interviewer training for field interviewers from all three sites was held before the project start and periodically throughout the course of the study. An overview of the research project, interviewing techniques, and review and

---

[2] In addition, we added a comparison group of nonpatients at the Pittsburgh site 1 year after data collection for the patient study had begun. This group was composed of people living in the neighborhoods in which the patients resided after hospital discharge. These community members were interviewed once about their behavior, including violence, in the past 10 weeks. Comparisons of the prevalence and characteristics of violence by the discharged patients and by their neighbors are reported in Steadman et al. (1998).

training on all the instruments was included. Interviewers participated in practice interviews with one another and were observed and critiqued. Large group discussion was important to ensure the standardization of interviewing objectives across sites. Videotapes that focused on specific components of the research instrument, such as the SIDP and Hare Psychopathy Checklist: Screening Version (Hare PCL:SV), were viewed. Clinically trained interviewers received additional training on psychiatric symptomatology (including delusions and hallucinations) and administration of the clinical instruments including observation and practice.

Additional training focused on the selection and replacement of collateral informants and administration of the collateral interview, with special attention to confidentiality issues that arise with multiple informants. All interviewers received numerous written and videotaped training materials in addition to the project-wide meetings.

Initial reliability studies took place during the spring and summer of 1992. As part of these studies, each interviewer videotaped five interviews with patients using the Baseline Interview they would be administering, and these interviews were circulated and coded in a systematic fashion among all the interviewers. This data set of 385 coded Baseline Research Interviews and 76 Baseline Clinical Interviews was analyzed to identify any additional training needs. Separate reliability studies for portions of the follow-up instrument and for the clinical portions of the interview to be administered in the community follow-up interviews (delusions, hallucinations, psychopathology, and functioning) were also conducted. Interrater reliability analyses for all key variables yielded excellent kappa coefficients on almost all data items collected (alpha >.80). Some modifications in scoring and additional training were performed when reliability results were unacceptable. The kappa coefficients for the violence screening sections of the instrument ranged from .85 to .98, well above the accepted .80 standard.

Violence and Safety Precautions

Although the extent of the ethical and legal duty to protect research subjects from self-harm and third parties and research staff from violence committed by subjects is unclear (Appelbaum & Rosenbaum, 1989), a series of safety procedures were incorporated into the study. What should research staff do if they believed that a subject would be imminently violent to self or others? The ethical and legal duty to protect subjects and third parties had to be balanced against the ethical and legal obligation to maintain subjects' confidentiality. Guidelines for action when interviewers suspected that violence to self or others was imminent were prepared at each site. Interviewers relayed information to senior staff, who ensured that it was reviewed by the site director and a clinical consultant. This "chain of command" and the hierarchy of interventions available (ranging from suggesting that the patient contact his or her therapist to independently contacting the patient's therapist or the police) — specified in writing in advance of any subject interviews — provided the framework for dealing with potentially dangerous situations as they arose. In addition, specific procedures were developed to protect the research interviewers, including staff training, case screening, and precautions to foster a secure interviewing environment. For a full discussion of the legal and ethical issues in conducting this research, see Monahan, Appelbaum, Mulvey, Robbins, and Lidz (1994).

DATA COLLECTION

Patient Sample

Admissions were sampled from acute inpatient facilities at the three sites used in the pilot study: Western Psychiatric Institute and Clinic (Pittsburgh, PA); Western Missouri Mental Health Center (Kansas City, MO); Worcester State Hospital and the University of Massachusetts Medical Center (Worcester, MA). Western Psychiatric Institute and Clinic (WPIC) is a university-based specialty hospital, Western Missouri Mental Health Center (WMMHC) is a regional mental health center, Worcester State Hospital (WSH) is one of first state mental hospitals in the United States, and the University of Massachusetts Medical Center (UMMC) is a teaching hospital and serves the mental and physical health needs of the surrounding community. UMMC was added as a recruitment site after hospital admissions at WSH dropped from 3.2 admits to 1.7 per day midway through the enrollment period.

Selection criteria for research subjects were (1) civil admissions; (2) age between 18 and 40 years; (3) ability to speak English; (4) white or African-American ethnicity (or Hispanic in Worcester only); and (5) a chart diagnosis of schizophrenia, schizophreniform, schizoaffective, depression, dysthymia, mania, brief reactive psychosis, delusional disorder, alcohol or drug abuse or dependence, or a personality disorder. Eligible patients were grouped according to age, gender, and race to maintain a consistent distribution of these characteristics across sites. These quota sample distributions were developed based on a power analysis that took into account the characteristics of admissions at the three sites and the prevalence of violence reported by subjects in the pilot study for this project. The mean time between hospital admission and approach by the research interviewer for consent to participate in the study was 4.5 days. Eligible subjects were excluded if they had been hospitalized for 21 days or more before being approached.

Hospital Data Collection

Descriptors on the patients admitted to the acute units were recorded at least twice a week, often daily, and entered into a computerized database for sampling according to age, gender, and race. Cases selected for study were approached by a research interviewer; most were approached within 4 days of their admission to the hospital after clearance to approach had been obtained from the hospital staff. To supplement information from the interviews, additional information regarding discharge diagnosis, length of hospitalization, and history of prior violence were abstracted from the patients' charts upon their discharge. To obtain information on possible sample bias, similar chart information was collected for a random sample of patients (approximately 1000 at each site) who were eligible for the study but not enrolled. A full discussion of all procedures can be found in Steadman et al. (1998).

Hospital data collection lasted about 2 hours and was conducted in two parts: (1) an interview by the research interviewer to obtain data on demographic and historical factors and (2) an interview by a research clinician (Ph.D. or MA/MSW) to confirm the chart diagnosis using the DSM-III-R Checklist (or to confirm a personality disorder using the Structured Interview for DSM-III-R Personality when no eligible Axis I diagnosis was present). Checklist diagnoses corresponded to a chart diagnosis in 85.7% of the cases.

Discrepant diagnoses were resolved by a consultant psychiatrist at each site. Patients remaining in the hospital for more than 145 days were dropped from the study (n = 3).

Postdischarge Data Collection

Patients were recontacted in the community by the research interviewers and interviewed up to five times (every 10 weeks) over 1 year from the date of discharge. Interviews were usually conducted by the research interviewer who had previously interviewed the patient in the hospital. Patient interviews were in person (89%) or by telephone (11%). All interviews took place with as much privacy as possible in order to eliminate bias in reporting due to the presence of other persons during the interview. Interviews were tape recorded for quality control and to clarify coding at a later time. Patients were paid $10 per interview ($15 for the final interview) for their participation in the study. Field interviewers invested large blocks of time in locating and securing follow-up interviews with discharged patients. Sites were provided with a "minimum acceptable contact" list itemizing the required attempts to contact a patient that had to be conducted before a patient was considered lost for the interview. Attempted contacts included phone calls or letters, visits to last known residences, and inquiries to relatives, local hospitals, jails, and shelters. The average number of contacts to locate a case was seven for the first follow-up interview and decreased to five for the fifth follow-up interview for those subjects who were located. Time from first contact to interview completion ranged across follow ups from 10.3 days in Pittsburgh to 16.0 days in Worcester.

Collaterals

Collateral interviews were conducted for each of the five community follow-up interviews for the 1000 patients being studied. The collateral informants were interviewed (in person, 45%; by telephone, 55%) on the same schedule as the patients. During each follow-up interview, a patient was asked to nominate as a collateral the person who was most familiar with his or her behavior in the community. If the nominee did not have at least weekly contact with the patient, the interviewer suggested a more appropriate person based on a review of the subject's social network data. Collaterals were most often family members (47.1%), but were also friends (23.9%), professionals (13.9%), significant others (12.4%), or others (e.g., co-workers, 2.7%). The collaterals were interviewed regarding the subject's violent behavior and the circumstances associated with it, the subject's level of functioning, and the subject's social support networks. Collaterals were paid for their participation at the same rate as the patients. Special efforts were made to ensure the confidentiality of the data obtained from collaterals, and in no case was this information shared with the patients (or vice versa).

Originally, the study design called for conducting collateral interviews after we had successfully completed the subject interview. This was because we wanted to confirm that the collateral was still a knowledgeable and appropriate informant and wanted to be careful not to violate the wishes of the subject should he or she no longer want to participate in the study (and therefore no longer want us to interview the collateral). That design decision was modified during data collection so that in cases where the subject had not refused to participate, but rather could not be located or scheduled for an interview during the appropriate time frame, we attempted to complete a collateral interview. We did not attempt to contact a collateral once the subject had withdrawn from the study.

Hospital and Arrest Records

Rehospitalization and arrest records provided the third source of information about the patients' behavior in the community. During the follow-up interviews, patients were asked whether they had been readmitted to a psychiatric facility. If a patient reported being readmitted, the hospital was contacted to obtain information regarding the rehospitalization, including dates of hospitalization, diagnosis, reasons for admission, and any reference to violence in the community. Records for any additional hospitalizations at the hospital from which the subject was recruited were also collected. After obtaining the subjects' informed consent, arrest records were obtained at the end of the 1 year follow-up period. These records contained complete adult arrest histories, as well as arrests that occurred during each follow-up period.

Violence Coding and Reconciliation

Subjects and collaterals were asked whether the subject had engaged in several categories of aggressive behavior in the past 10 weeks before their admission to the hospital and then during each follow-up interview. Each respondent was asked first whether the patient had particular violent acts (e.g., hitting, slapping) done to them during the prior 2 months and then was asked whether the patient had done these acts to others. The list of violent acts was adapted from the Conflicts Tactics Scale (Gelles & Straus, 1988) and had been used successfully in prior research with discharged psychiatric patients in the community (Mulvey, Shaw, & Lidz, 1994). The interviewer then reviewed all of the positive responses and ascertained whether these were separate incidents of violence or whether some of the violent acts noted had occurred during a single incident.

If there was more than one type of violent act that occurred in a single incident, the incident was coded as involving the most serious type of act. Information about the violent events reported by subjects and collaterals included detailed descriptions of each violent incident (i.e., in terms of date, incident location, victim relationships, seriousness and type of injury to victim, and whether a weapon was used).

For incidents involving weapons or injury, a detailed narrative report was also obtained. The respondent was then asked to provide additional details regarding each incident, for example, whether certain conditions held at the time of the incident (e.g., whether the patient had been drinking).

The reconciliation of all these data sources was conducted at the coordinating study site, PRA. All available sources of information were compared by research associates, and a determination was made about whether a particular incident occurred and what most likely occurred during the incident. These research associates followed a set of explicit decision making guidelines (available from the authors) for determining whether an incident occurred and which account of the incident (or which combination of accounts) to accept as a valid representation of the incident. Acts reported by any information source were reviewed by two independent coders to obtain a single reconciled report of violence.

Once the reports were independently coded by the two coders, the reports were compared and any differences resolved by a third coder. For example, subject self-reports of violence, and arrests for violence, were accepted when they were available. Collateral reports of violence were accepted if the collateral was present at the incident or had heard about the incident directly from the subject. Collateral reports were not accepted if the collateral only had heard about an incident from a third party. A hierarchical set of rules for this reconciliation procedure was developed.

Subject and collateral sources were rated by project interviewers in terms of their honesty in reporting — on a five-point Likert scale ranging from 1 = Honest to 5 = Untruthful. These sources were also rated in terms of whether they were perceived as over- or underreporting violence or accurately reporting violence. Matching discrete incidents across information sources was accomplished by using the date, victim, type of violence, description of the incident, and nature of injury. This produced a final reconciled account of violence and other aggressive acts.

DATA MANAGEMENT

Tracking

The tracking database developed for the MacArthur Violence Risk Assessment Study played an integral role in the data collection process. The tracking database served twofold purposes: (1) it allowed each site to systematically track and monitor the status of its enrolled (and nonenrolled) clients, and (2) it enabled the coordinating center to have a uniform set of variables from each site, which facilitates verifying and cleaning the tracking database. Moreover, it provided the sites — and the coordinating center — with a mechanism for identifying which subjects were due for interviews. The database enabled PRA to ensure that all completed interviews were indeed received for processing and enabled the sites to generate lists of all upcoming interviews on or before the targeted completion date. The extract feature conveniently allowed the sites to regularly update the coordinating center on the following: (1) all subjects enrolled, (2) all subjects interviewed, and (3) those scheduled for interviews. A monthly extract was submitted, via diskette or E-mail, to update the coordinating center. Another feature of the tracking database allowed the sites to produce and print four different types of reports, which included (1) a list of all clients and their enrollment status by ID and assigned interviewer; (2) a list of only enrolled clients by ID and name; (3) individual interview schedules for each respective interviewer; and (4) an overall schedule report, listing the interviewer and the status of all impending interviews. The former reports are useful for seeing the differences between the number of enrolled versus nonenrolled subjects, while the latter reports serve the practical needs of the site, enabling them to print out a weekly list of those clients scheduled to be interviewed by each interviewer.

Quality Control

All data collected at the sites were sent for central quality control and data processing. Interview forms, contact logs, and audiotapes were shipped throughout the data collection period. Data were sorted, logged in, and filed numerically by unique study identification numbers. A forms tracking program (SPSS data entry) was used to monitor the forms and tapes that were shipped to PRA. Periodically, the SPSS forms tracking program was linked with the tracking program discussed above to create a comprehensive list of all ID numbers and the status of all forms and tapes. This was sent to each site regularly as an additional way to check on materials and reconcile each site's records with central reports.

All forms were reviewed by PRA staff. Question by question, the coding was checked for completion, accuracy in skip patterns, internal consistency, and valid response codes. Because of the inevitable permutations that arise when conducting personal interviews, the field interviewers had been instructed to write notes about any subject responses or additional information that did not easily fit the response categories. This information was used to make coding decisions.

Although there were many examples of the benefits of a centralized data cleaning and data management function, the residence grids on the follow-up interview illustrate the level of form review required. Because time spent in the community is a key variable to the research project, the number of days during each follow-up period had to be carefully accounted for. It was important to check the number of days that the subject reported living in the community (in his or her own residence, a group home, a shelter, or on the streets) as opposed to being out of the community (in a hospital, a residential detox facility, or in jail). The inherent difficulties of memory recall were compounded by the often present psychiatric symptomatology of the study population. The subjects often reported moving, going in and out of hospitals, being on the streets, or simply not recalling where they were during a 2.5 month period. Constructing the residence grid became a complex task. Reference dates were calculated to find the number of days in each follow-up period, and then residence grid reports were checked to ensure that all days were accounted for. The interview schedule repeatedly posed questions about various treatments, psychiatric hospitalizations, detox programs, or time in jail; it was important to check for the potential problem of the subject reporting the same treatment and/or hospital stay more than once and the interviewer over-coding the time spent out of the community.

A key task of debriefing was to check each question that was coded for time out of the community against all other similar questions and to reconcile that compilation of days with the number of days that was reported on the residence grid. All incomplete (missing) or questionable data on the grids and elsewhere on the forms were completed by listening to the audiotapes or returning the forms to the sites for completion.

Code books were created for all instruments and data entry programs. Each interviewer had access to these code books to use as a primary reference manual for coding decisions. Coding decisions were made at PRA in response to a number of issues that arose from data collection. Most of these coding decisions made after the onset of data collection related to open-ended questions. After the responses to the questions asked during the early stages of data collection were reviewed, the responses were compiled and grouped in coding categories. These coding changes were dated and transmitted to the interviewers at each site in order to avoid potential discrepancies among interviewers.

Data entry and verification were performed for all forms received. The data entry program provided another level of data quality checks with programmed range and skip rules. All data were checked with statistical analyses for outliers and other data problems once data entry was completed. The data set was created and stored in many files due to the amount of data collected (over 25,000 items in the data set for each subject), which necessitated considerable file merging and file management.

RESULTS

Enrollment and Retention

By October 1994, 1136 subjects had been enrolled into the MacArthur Violence Risk Assessment Study and had completed baseline hospital interviews. Subject enrollment ceased at this point.

During the study period, 12,873 persons were admitted to the facilities participating in the research, of whom 7740 met our eligibility criteria. We approached a stratified sample of 1695 of these patients for consent to take part in the study. The refusal rate was 29.0% (n = 492). The final sample given a hospital interview was 1136, because 67 of the 1203 subjects who consented to participate were released before they could be interviewed. The median length of hospitalization for enrolled patients at the three sites was 9.0 days.

Of the subjects interviewed in the hospital, 45 were unavailable for follow-up interviews in the community (34 because they dropped out of the research before the first follow-up interview, 8 because they had spent no time in the community during the first follow-up period, and 3 because their hospital stay exceeded the study's maximum of 145 days). All subjects who did not complete at least one of the first three follow-up interviews in the community were dropped from the study for future follow-up interviews. Data collection continued for the subjects who remained in the study. Attempts were made to interview these subjects and their collaterals in the community for the year following release.

We obtained at least one follow-up interview in the community for 83.7% of the enrolled patients. Table A.1 presents the percentage of subjects and collaterals who completed various numbers of follow-up interviews. Three or more follow-up interviews were obtained for 72.0% of the patients and 77.3% of the collaterals, and all five follow-up interviews were obtained for 49.6% of the patients and 44.7% of the collaterals.

TABLE A.1. Completed Follow-Up Interviews for Subjects and Collaterals

No. of Follow-Up Interviews	Subject Interviews (n = 1136)		Collateral Interviews (n = 951)	
	No.	%	No.	%
1 or more	951	83.7	897	94.3
2 or more	893	78.6	838	88.1
3 or more	818	72.0	735	77.3
4 or more	731	64.3	609	64.0
All 5	564	49.6	425	44.7

Demographic and diagnostic characteristics of the sample of eligible admissions, the patients who refused to participate, the baseline sample, patients lost to follow up, and the follow-up sample are reported in Table A.2. There it can be seen that patients who consented to participate were significantly younger, less likely to have a chart diagnosis of schizophrenia, and more likely to have chart diagnoses of alcohol/drug abuse and personality disorder than patients who refused to participate. Compared with enrolled patients lost to follow-up study, patients in the follow-up sample were significantly more likely to have a chart diagnosis of bipolar disorder, less likely to have a chart diagnosis or a chart history of alcohol/drug abuse, less likely to have a legal status of gravely disabled, and less likely to have a chart history of violence toward family members or others. As we stated in Steadman et al. (1998):

> An inevitable limitation of research in this area is that patient refusal or attrition can compromise the representativeness of the sample studied. Some of the biases we observed are in the direction of patients in our sample being more likely to be violent than other eligible patients (e.g., patients who consented were younger than patients who refused) and other biases are in the direction of patients in our sample being less likely to be violent than other eligible patients (e.g., patients followed-up were less likely to have a documented history of violence than patients lost to follow-up). It is impossible to estimate the precise effect of these countervailing biases on the results. (pp. 400–401)

TABLE A.2. Sample Description (%)

	Sample of Eligible Admissions (n = 7740)	Refused to Participate (n = 492)	Baseline Sample (n = 1136)	Lost to Follow-Up (n = 185)	Follow-Up Sample (n = 951)
Demographics					
Gender					
Male	57.6	60.4	58.7	64.3	57.6
Female	42.4	39.6	41.3	35.7	42.4
Race					
White	55.9	69.7	69.1	70.8	68.8
African-American	42.6	27.8	29.0	29.2	29.0
Hispanic	1.5	2.4	1.8	0.0	2.2
Age					
18–24	19.7	19.1*	24.7	30.3	23.7
25–40	80.3	80.9*	75.3	69.7	76.3
Chart admission diagnosis					
Depression	20.3	20.7	22.8	18.4	23.7
Bipolar	27.8	32.1	35.5	26.5**	37.2
Schizophrenia	26.0	43.7***	20.0	17.8	20.4
Alcohol/drug	59.3	42.1***	57.7	64.9*	56.4
Personality disorder	36.6	25.8***	37.4	39.5	37.0
Organic disorder	10.2	8.9	9.1	7.6	9.4
Any chart diagnosis with comorbid alcohol or drug diagnosis	37.6	32.7	36.2	33.0	36.8
Chart history of alcohol or drug abuse	83.9§	NA	72.9	82.1**	71.4
Prior hospitalizations: at least one	67.7§	NA	72.1	68.5	72.7
Legal status					
Involuntary	34.7§	39.2	41.9	40.5	42.0
Danger to self	27.8§	NA	39.0	38.1	39.1
Danger to others	13.8§	NA	14.1	13.6	14.2
Gravely disabled	6.0§	NA	2.2	6.3***	1.4
Chart History of violence¶					
Violent/aggressive toward family	29.1§	NA	28.9	42.7***	26.5
Violent/aggressive towards others	47.3§	NA	40.9	54.2**	38.6

§Data come from a sample of 3095 cases across the three sites weighted by site.

¶Violent/aggressive toward family members and toward others not mutually exclusive.

Footnotes indicate significant difference for either (1) a comparison of those who Refused to Participate with those enrolled in the Baseline sample or (2) a comparison of those Lost to Follow-up with those in the Follow-up sample:

* p <.05 ** p <.01 *** p <.001.

CONCLUSIONS

A great deal of time and resources were devoted to the collection of a comprehensive data set for use in the MacArthur Violence Risk Assessment Study. This book highlights findings from these data on the level and type of violence we observed, on the relationship between key risk factors and violence, and on how risk factors were combined to result in a new tool for violence risk assessment.

APPENDIX B

TABLE B1. Risk Factors and Associations with Violence During the First Two Follow-up Periods*

Risk Factor	Reference	Pearson R	Unstandardized Odds Ratio	Standardized Odds Ratio	p value
Personal Domain					
Sex—Male		.08	1.51	1.23	.017
Age		−.07	0.97	0.83	.027
Race—White		−.12	0.54	0.75	.000
Verbal IQ†		−.11	0.98	0.74	.001
Ever Married		.01	1.03	1.01	.873
Hare PCL:SV > 12†	Hart, Cox, & Hare (1995a)	.26	4.05	1.79	.000
Novaco Anger— Behavior	Novaco (1994)	.16	1.06	1.52	.000
Novaco Anger— Cognitive		.11	1.04	1.24	.012
Novaco Anger— Arousal		.09	1.04	1.28	.004
Novaco Anger— Intensity		.08	1.02	1.25	.011
Barrett Impulsiveness, Motor	Barratt (1994)	.07	1.02	1.20	.029
Barrett Impulsiveness, Nonplanning		.05	1.02	1.15	.102
Barrett Impulsiveness, Cognitive		.05	1.02	1.13	.162

(continued)

TABLE B1. Risk Factors and Associations with Violence During the First Two Follow-up Periods*—Continued

Risk Factor	Reference	Pearson R	Unstandardized Odds Ratio	Standardized Odds Ratio	p value
Historical Domain					
Years of Education		−.11	0.88	0.75	.001
Socioeconomic Status†	Holingshead & Redlich (1958)	.05	1.01	1.15	.107
Employed		−.05	0.76	0.87	.108
Age at First Hospitalization		−.04	0.99	0.90	.196
No. of Prior Hospitalizations		−.03	0.99	0.91	.326
Involuntary Legal Status		.11	1.78	1.31	.001
Recent Violent Behavior		.14	2.32	1.37	.000
Adult Arrest—Seriousness		.25	2.04	1.83	.000
Adult Arrest—Frequency		.24	1.60	1.85	.000
Any Arrest Person Crime†	Official Report	.13	2.11	1.36	.000
Any Arrest Other Crime†	Official Report	.11	1.80	1.33	.001
Sexually Abused Before Age 20		−.03	0.85	0.92	.335
Seriousness of Abuse as Child		.14	1.51	1.50	.000
Frequency of Abuse as Child		.12	1.25	1.40	.000
Father Ever Used Drugs		.16	2.40	1.41	.000
Father Ever Arrested		.15	1.79	1.43	.000
Father Ever Excess Drinking		.11	1.87	1.36	.001
Father Ever Admitted to Psych Hosp		.02	1.14	1.05	.552
Lived with Father to Age 15		−.09	0.63	0.79	.006
Mother Ever Used Drugs		.05	1.54	1.12	.000
Mother Ever Arrested		.05	1.24	1.11	.168
Mother Ever Excess Drinking		.06	1.41	1.16	.072
Mother Ever Admitted to Psych Hosp		−.02	0.92	0.95	.585

(continued)

Risk Factor	Reference	Pearson R	Unstandardized Odds Ratio	Standardized Odds Ratio	p value
Lived with Mother to Age 15		−.06	0.72	0.87	.091
Parents Ever Fought with Each Other		.06	1.13	1.15	.098
Parents Ever Fought with Others		.03	1.10	1.08	.330
Any Head Injury— Loss of Consciousness	Silver & Caton (1989)	.10	1.69	1.30	.002
Any Head Injury— No Loss of Consciousness	Silver & Caton (1989)	.06	1.43	1.18	.055
Self-Harm Thoughts		.02	1.13	1.06	.473
Self-Harm Attempt		−.03	0.77	0.93	.387
Attempt to Kill Self		.01	1.08	1.03	.726
Contextual Domain					
Living in Private Residence		−.05	0.70	0.88	.105
Homeless		.05	1.66	1.12	.132
Living Alone		−.07	0.61	0.82	.038
Perceived Stress†	Cohen, Kamarck, & Mermelstein (1983)	.08	1.54	1.23	.019
Social Networks (Estroff & Zimmer, 1994)					
No. of People in Social Network†		−.02	0.99	0.96	.596
% MH Prof in Social Network†		−.10	0.13	0.74	.004
% Family in Social Network†		.01	1.15	1.03	.683
No. of Negative Persons in Social Network†		.07	1.14	1.20	.026
No. of Positive and Material Supporters†		−.07	0.91	0.83	.030
Avg No. of Mentions per Negative Person†		.06	1.21	1.16	.067

(continued)

TABLE B1. Risk Factors and Associations with Violence During the First Two Follow-up Periods* — Continued

Risk Factor	Reference	Pearson R	Unstandardized Odds Ratio	Standardized Odds Ratio	p value
Avg No. of Mentions per Pos/Mat Person†		−.03	0.75	0.94	.424
Frequency of Social Network Contact†		−.03	0.88	0.93	.394
Duration of Social Network Contact†		.02	1.05	1.04	.630
Clinical Domain					
Chart Antisocial Personality Disorder		.19	3.11	1.48	.000
DSM-III-R Checklist (Janca & Helzer, 1990)					
Major Disorder, No Substance Disorder		−.19	0.34	0.59	.000
Major Disorder and Substance Disorder		.08	1.47	1.21	.021
Substance Disorder, No Major Disorder		.15	2.47	1.38	.000
Drug or alcohol		.18	2.74	1.65	.000
Drug		.17	2.37	1.51	.000
Alcohol		.14	2.08	1.44	.000
Schizophrenia		−.12	0.38	0.69	.001
Mania		−.04	0.74	0.89	.214
Depression		−.02	0.92	0.96	.630
Other Psychosis		.00	1.00	1.00	1.000
Personality Disorder Only		.02	1.46	1.06	.471
Brief Psychiatric Rating Scale (BPRS) (Overall, 1988)					
Total Score†		−.04	0.99	0.91	.251
Activation Subscale†		−.08	0.87	0.78	.011
Hostility Subscale†		.08	1.06	1.21	.020
Anergia Subscale†		−.07	0.94	0.82	.037
Thought Disturbance Subscale†		−.06	0.96	0.84	.052
Anxiety/Depression Subscale†		.01	1.00	1.02	.848
Global Assessment of Functioning	American Psychiatric Association (1989)	−.05	0.99	0.89	.171

(continued)

TABLE B1.—Continued

Risk Factor	Reference	Pearson R	Unstandardized Odds Ratio	Standardized Odds Ratio	p value
Activities of Daily Living		−.01	0.99	0.98	.791
Delusions (Appelbaum, Robbins, & Roth, 1999)					
Any Delusions†		−.06	0.74	0.87	.116
Persecutory		−.07	0.61	0.82	.029
Grandiose		−.01	0.90	0.97	.692
Body/Mind Control		−.09	0.49	0.77	.009
Thought Broadcasting		−.05	0.60	0.86	.130
Religious		−.08	0.37	0.76	.021
Jealousy		−.02	0.02	0.84	.696
Guilt		−.03	0.56	0.91	.348
Somatic		−.03	0.61	0.92	.433
Influence on Others		−.03	0.02	0.81	.632
Threat/Control Override		−.10	0.76	0.69	.003
Other		−.04	0.78	0.94	.467
Violent Fantasies (Grisso et al., 2000)					
Any		.13	1.94	1.35	.000
Frequent		.13	2.23	1.32	.000
Recent Onset		.07	1.74	1.17	.038
Same Target		.03	1.26	1.07	.368
Focus Same Person		.10	1.91	1.25	.003
Escalating Harm		.13	2.80	1.29	.000
While with Target		.12	2.08	1.32	.000
Frequent, Not Escalating, not with Target		−.01	0.87	0.97	.772
Frequent, Escalating, Not with Target		.09	4.46	1.18	.010
Frequent, Not Escalating, with Target		.08	1.94	1.18	.021
Frequent, Escalating, with Target		.10	3.49	1.21	.004
Not Frequent, Not Escalating, Not with Target		.13	0.50	0.75	.000
Any Hallucinations		.02	1.12	1.06	.517
Command Hallucinations		.06	1.43	1.14	.088

(continued)

TABLE B1. Risk Factors and Associations with Violence During the First Two Follow-up Periods* —Continued

Risk Factor	Reference	Pearson R	Unstandardized Odds Ratio	Standardized Odds Ratio	p value
Present at Time of Admission (Record Review)					
Substance Abuse		.14	2.01	1.41	.000
Paranoia		−.09	0.39	0.74	.006
Delusions		−.09	0.45	0.76	.007
Decompensation		−.09	0.55	0.78	.010
Violence		.09	1.97	1.21	.010
Hallucinations		−.07	0.62	0.82	.027
Bizarre Behavior		−.07	0.41	0.79	.040
Med Nonadherence		−.07	0.54	0.82	.048
Aggressive (Nonviolent)		.06	1.44	1.16	.054
Anxiety		−.05	0.65	0.86	.103
Suicide Attempt		.05	1.31	1.12	.161
Mania		−.04	0.57	0.88	.200
Personal Problems		.03	1.17	1.08	.355
Evaluation		.03	1.25	1.06	.427
Other		−.03	0.66	0.93	.449
Medication Change		−.02	0.75	0.95	.603
Unable to Care for Self		.02	1.29	1.04	.623
Suicide Threat		−.01	0.94	0.97	.737
Property Damage		−.01	0.90	0.98	.841
Court Order		−.01	0.92	0.98	.845
Depression		−.003	0.99	0.99	.934
Drug Use					
Any Drug		.12	1.89	1.35	.000
Cocaine		.11	1.95	1.28	.001
Alcohol		.10	1.66	1.29	.003
Other		.08	3.46	.17	.015
Marijuana		.04	1.31	1.11	.179
Stimulants		.04	1.82	1.08	.267
Sedatives		.03	1.40	1.08	.311
Opiates		.04	1.52	1.09	.244
Mini Mental Status†	Folstein, Folstein, & McHugh (1975)	.02	1.13	1.06	.508
Perceived Coercion at Admission†	Gardner et al. (1993)	.03	1.04	1.08	.357

*Measures with no reference were obtained by using project instruments and are available from the authors.

†Omitted from the "clinically feasible" analyses.

REFERENCES

American Bar Association. (1998). *National benchbook on psychiatric and psychological evidence and testimony.* Washington, DC: American Bar Association.

American Psychiatric Association. (1983). Guidelines for legislation on the psychiatric hospitalization of adults. *American Journal of Psychiatry, 140,* 672–679.

American Psychiatric Association (1989). *Diagnostic and Statistical Manual of Mental Disorders* (3rd ed, Rev). Washington, DC: American Psychiatric Association.

Anderson, E. (1990). *Streetwise: Race, class, and change in an urban community.* Chicago: IL: University of Chicago Press.

Appelbaum, P. (1988). The new preventive detention: Psychiatry's problematic responsibility for the control of violence. *American Journal of Psychiatry, 145,* 779–785.

Appelbaum, P. (1994). *Almost a revolution: Mental health law and the limits of change.* New York: Oxford University Press.

Appelbaum, P., Robbins, P., & Monahan, J. (2000). Violence and delusions: Data from the MacArthur Violence Risk Assessment Study. *American Journal of Psychiatry, 157,* 566–572.

Appelbaum, P. S., Robbins, P. C., & Roth, L. H. (1999). A dimensional approach to the assessment of delusions. *American Journal of Psychiatry, 156,* 1938–1943.

Appelbaum, P., & Rosenbaum, A. (1989). *Tarasoff* and the researcher: Does the duty to protect apply in the research setting? *American Psychologist, 44,* 885–894.

Arseneault, L., Moffitt, T., Caspi, A., Taylor, P., & Silva, P. (2000). Mental disorders and violence in a total birth cohort: Results from the Dunedin Study. *Archives of General Psychiatry, 57,* 979–986.

Bandura, A. (1973). *Aggression: A social learning analysis.* Englewood Cliffs, NJ: Prentice Hall.

Banks, S., Robbins, P., Silver, E., Vesselinov, R., Steadman, H., Monahan, J., Mulvey, E., Appelbaum, P., Grisso, T., & Roth, L. (in press). A multiple models approach to violence risk assessment among people with mental disorder. *Criminal Justice and Behavior.*

Barratt, E. (1994). Impulsiveness and aggression. In J. Monahan, & H. Steadman, (Eds.), *Violence and mental disorder: Developments in risk assessment* (pp. 61–79). Chicago: University of Chicago Press.

Baxter, R. (1997). Violence in schizophrenia and the syndrome of disorganization. *Criminal Behaviour and Mental Health, 7,* 131–139.

Belfrage, H. (1998). A ten-year follow-up of criminality in Stockholm mental patients. *British Journal of Criminology, 38,* 145–155.

Berger, J., & Gross, J. (1998). Yale graduate is charged with killing his fiancée. *New York Times,* June 19, p. A29.

Binder, R., & McNiel, D. (1999). Contemporary practices in managing acutely violent patients in 20 psychiatric emergency rooms. *Psychiatric Services, 50,* 1553–1554.

Blackburn, R. (1988). On moral judgments and personality disorders: The myth of the psychopathic personality revisited. *British Journal of Psychiatry, 153,* 505–512.

Blackburn, R. (1998). Psychopathy and personality disorder: Implications of interpersonal theory. In D. Cooke, A. Forth, & R. Hare, (Eds.), *Psychopathy: Theory, research, and implications for society* (pp. 269–301). Dordrecht, the Netherlands: Kluwer Academic.

Bloom, J., Mueser, K. & Müller-Isberner, R. (2000). Treatment implications of the antecedents of criminality and violence in schizophrenia and major affective disorders. In S. Hodgins (Ed.), *Effective prevention of crime and violence among the mentally ill* (pp. 145–170). Dordrecht, the Netherlands: Kluwer Academic.

Blumenthal, S., & Lavender, T. (2000). *Violence and mental disorder.* Hereford, England: The Zito Trust.

Blumstein, A., Cohen, J., Roth, J., & Visher, C. (1986). *Criminal careers and "career criminals."* Washington, DC: National Academy Press.

Bonnie, R., & Monahan, J. (Eds.). (1997). *Mental disorder, work disability, and the law.* Chicago: University of Chicago Press.

Bonta, J., Law, M., & Hanson, K. (1998). The prediction of criminal and violent recidivism among mentally disordered offenders: A meta-analysis. *Psychological Bulletin, 123,* 123–142.

Borum, R. (1996). Improving the clinical practice of violence risk assessment: Technology, guidelines, and training. *American Psychologist, 51,* 945, 948.

Breiman, L., Friedman, J., Olshen, R., & Stone, C. (1984). *Classification and regression trees.* Pacific Grove, CA: Wadsworth and Brooks/Cole.

Brennan, P., Mednick, S., & Hodgins, S. (2000). Major mental disorders and criminal violence in a Danish birth cohort. *Archives of General Psychiatry, 57,* 494–500.

Buchanan A. (1999). Risk and dangerousness. *Psychological Medicine, 29,* 465–473.

Burgess, E. (1928). Factors determining success or failure on parole. In A. A. Bruce (Ed.), *The workings on the indeterminate sentence law and the parole system in Illinois.* Springfield: Illinois State Board of Parole.

Carson, D. (1997). A risk management approach to legal decision-making about "dangerous" people. In R. Baldwin (Ed.), *Law and uncertainty: Risk and legal processes* (pp. 255–269). London: Klumer Law international.

Carter, G., & Polger, P. (1986). *A 20-year summary of National Weather Service verification results for temperature and precipitation.* (Technical Memorandum NWS FCST 31). Washington, DC: National Oceanic and Atmospheric Administration.

Champion, D. (1994). *Measuring offender risk: A criminal justice sourcebook.* Westport, CT: Greenwood Press.

Cleckley, H. (1941). *The mask of sanity.* St. Louis: Mosby.

Climent, C. E., Rollins, A., Ervin, F. R., & Plutchik, R. (1973). Epidemiological studies of women prisoners I: Medical and psychiatric variables related to violent behavior. *American Journal of Psychiatry, 130,* 985–990.

Cocozza, J., & Steadman, H. (1976). The failure of psychiatric predictions of dangerousness: Clear and convincing evidence. *Rutgers Law Review, 29,* 1084–1101.

Cohen, S., Kamarck, T., & Mermelstein, R. (1983). A global measure of perceived stress. *Journal of Health and Social Behavior, 24,* 385–396.

Convit, A., Jaeger, J., Lin, S., Meisner, M., & Volavka, J. (1988). Predicting assaultiveness in psychiatric inpatients: A pilot study. *Hospital and Community Psychiatry, 39,* 429–434.

Cook, T., & Campbell, D. (1979). *Quasi-experimentation: Design and analysis issues for field settings.* Skokie, IL: Rand McNally.

Cooke, D., & Michie, C. (in press). Refining the construct of psychopathy: Towards a hierarchical model. *Psychological Assessment.*

Crowner, M. (Ed) (2000). *Understanding and treating violent psychiatric patients.* Washington, DC: American Psychiatric Press.

Dean, K., & Malamuth, N., (1997). Characteristics of men who aggress sexually and of men who imagine aggressing: Risk and moderating variables. *Journal of Personality and Social Psychology, 72*, 449–455.

Dennis, D., & Monahan, J. (Eds.). (1996). *Coercion and aggressive community treatment: A new frontier in mental health law.* New York: Plenum Publishing Corporation.

Douglas, K., Cox, D., & Webster, C. (1999). Violence risk assessment: Science and practice. *Legal and Criminological Psychology, 4*, 149–184.

Douglas, K., Ogloff, J., Nicholls, T., & Grant, I. (1999). Assessing risk for violence among psychiatric patients: The HCR-20 Violence Risk Assessment Scheme and the Psychopathy Checklist: Screening Version. *Journal of Consulting and Clinical Psychology, 67*, 917–930.

Douglas, K., & Webster, C. (1999). The HCR-20 violence risk assessment scheme: Concurrent validity in a sample of incarcerated offenders. *Criminal Justice and Behavior, 26*, 3–19.

Drake, R., Mercer-McFadden, C., Mueser, K., McHugo, G., & Bond, G. (1998). Review of integrated mental health and substance abuse treatment for patients with dual disorders. *Schizophrenia Bulletin, 24*, 589–608.

Earles, F., & Barnes, J. (1997). Understanding and preventing child abuse in urban settings. In McCord, J. (Ed.), *Violence and childhood in the inner city* (pp. 207–255). Cambridge: Cambridge University Press.

Efron, B. (1979). Bootstrap methods: Another look at the jackknife. *Annals of Mathematical Statistics, 7*, 1–26.

Elbogen, E. B., Mercado, C., Tomkins, A. J., & Scalora, M. J. (in press). Clinical practice and violence risk assessment: Availability of MacArthur risk factors. In D. Farrington, C. R. Hollin, & M. McMurran (Eds.), *Sex and violence: The psychology of crimes and risk assessment.* Reading, England: Harwood Academic.

Estroff, S., & Zimmer, C. (1994). Social networks, social support, and violence among persons with severe, persistent mental illness. In Monahan, J. & Steadman, H. (Eds.), *Violence and mental disorder: Developments in risk assessment* (pp. 259–295). Chicago: University of Chicago Press.

Estroff, S., Zimmer, C., Lachicotte, W., & Benoit, J. (1994). The influence of social networks and social support on violence by persons with serious mental illness. *Hospital and Community Psychiatry, 45*, 669–679.

First, M., Spitzer, R., Gibbon, M., Williams, J. (1999). *Computer-assisted SCID—Clinician version.* North Tonowanda, NY: Multi-Health Systems.

First, M., Williams, J., & Spitzer, R. (1998). *DTREE: The DSM-IV expert.* North Tonowanda, NY: Multi-Health Systems.

Folstein, M., Folstein, S., & McHugh, P. (1975). Mini-mental state: A practical method for grading the cognitive state of patients for the clinician. *Journal of Psychiatric Research, 12,* 189–198.

Garb, H. (1998). *Studying the clinician: Judgment research and psychological assessment.* Washington, DC: American Psychological Association.

Gardner, W., Hoge, S., Bennett, N., Roth, L., Lidz, C., Monahan, J., & Mulvey, E. (1993). Two scales for measuring patients' perceptions of coercion during hospital admission. *Behavioral Sciences and the Law, 20,* 307–321.

Gardner, W., Lidz, C., Mulvey, E., & Shaw, E. (1996a). A comparison of actuarial methods for identifying repetitively violent patients with mental illness. *Law and Human Behavior, 20,* 35–48.

Gardner, W., Lidz, C., Mulvey, E., & Shaw, E. (1996b). Clinical versus actuarial predictions of violence in patients with mental illnesses. *Journal of Consulting and Clinical Psychology, 64,* 602.

Gelles, R., & Straus, M. (1988). *Intimate violence: The causes and consequences of abuse in the American family.* New York: Simon & Schuster.

Gottfredson, S. D., & Gottfredson, D. M. (1980). Screening for risk: A comparison of methods. *Criminal Justice and Behavior, 7,* 315–330.

Greenfeld, L., & Snell, T. (1999). *Bureau of Justice Statistics special report: Women offenders.* Washington, DC: U. S. Department of Justice.

Greenwald, D., & Harder, D. (1997). Fantasies, coping behavior, and psychopathology. *Journal of Clinical Psychology, 53,* 91–97.

Grisso, T., & Appelbaum, P. (1998). *Assessing competence to consent to treatment: A guide for physicians and other health professionals.* New York: Oxford University Press.

Grisso, T., Davis, J., Vesselinov, R., Appelbaum, P., & Monahan, J. (2000). Violent thoughts and violent behavior following hospitalization for mental disorder. *Journal of Consulting and Clinical Psychology 68,* 388–398.

Grove, W., & Meehl, P. (1996). Comparative efficacy of informal (subjective, impressionistic) and formal (mechanical, algorithmic) prediction procedures: The clinical–statistical controversy. *Psychology, Public Policy, and Law, 2,* 293–323.

Grove, W., Zald, D., Lebow, B., Snitz, B., & Nelson, C. (2000). Clinical versus mechanical prediction: A meta-analysis. *Psychological Assessment, 12,* 19–30.

Grunwald, M. & Boodman, S. (1998). Weston case "fell through the cracks." *Washington Post,* July 28, p. A1.

Gunn, J. (1998). Psychopathy: An elusive concept with moral overtones. In T. Millon, E. Simonsen, M. Birket-Smith, & R. Davis, (Eds.), *Psychopathy: Antisocial, criminal, and violent behavior* (pp. 32–39). New York: Guilford Press.

Gunn, J. (2000). Future directions for treatment in forensic psychiatry. *British Journal of Psychiatry, 176,* 332–338.

Gutheil, T., & Appelbaum, P. (2000). *Clinical handbook of psychiatry and the law* (3rd ed.). Baltimore: Williams & Wilkins.

Hanson, R. (1998). What do we know about sex offender risk assessment? *Psychology, Public Policy, and Law, 4*, 50–72.

Hare, R. (1980). A research scale for the assessment of psychopathy in criminal populations. *Personality and Individual Differences, 1*, 111–119.

Hare, R. (1991). *The Hare Psychopathy Checklist—Revised.* Toronto: Multi-Health Systems.

Hare, R. (1996). Psychopathy: A clinical construct whose time has come. *Criminal Justice and Behavior, 23*, 25.

Hare, R. (1998). The Hare PCL-R: Some issues concerning its use and misuse. *Legal and Criminological Psychology, 2*, 99–119.

Hare, R. (1999). Psychopathy as a risk factor for violence. *Psychiatric Quarterly, 70*, 181–197.

Hare, R., Harpur, T., Hakistan, R., Forth, A., Hart, S., & Newman, J. (1990). The Revised Psychopathy Checklist: Reliability and factor structure. *Psychological Assessment: A Journal of Consulting and Clinical Psychology, 2*, 338–341.

Harpur, T., & Hare, R. (1994). The assessment of psychopathy as a function of age. *Journal of Abnormal Psychology, 103*, 604–609.

Harpur, T., Hare, R., & Hakistan, R. (1989). A two-factor conceptualization of psychopathy: Construct validity and implications for assessment. *Psychological Assessment: A Journal of Consulting and Clinical Psychology, 1*, 6–17.

Harris, G., Rice, M., & Cormier, C. (1991). Psychopathy and violent recidivism. *Law and Human Behavior, 15*, 625–637.

Harris, G., Rice, M. & Quinsey, V. (1993). Violent recidivism of mentally disordered offenders: The development of a statistical prediction instrument. *Criminal Justice and Behavior, 20*, 315.

Hart, S. (1998a). Psychopathy and risk for violence. In D. Cooke, A. Forth, & R. Hare, (Eds.), *Psychopathy: Theory, research, and implications for society* (pp. 355–373). Dordrecht, the Netherlands: Kluwer Academic.

Hart, S. (1998b). The role of psychopathy in assessing risk for violence: Conceptual and methodological issues. *Legal and Criminological Psychology, 3*, 121–137.

Hart, S., Cox, D., & Hare, R. (1995a). *The Hare Psychopathy Checklist: Screening Version.* Toronto: Multi-Health Systems.

Hart, S., Cox, D., & Hare, R. (1995b). *Manual for the Psychopathy Checklist: Screening Version (PCL:SV).* Toronto: Multi-Health Systems.

Hart, S., Hare, R., & Forth, A. (1994). Psychopathy as a risk marker for violence: Development and validation of a screening version of the Revised Psychopathy Checklist. In J. Monahan, & H. Steadman, (Eds.), *Violence and mental disorder:*

Developments in risk assessment (pp. 81–98). Chicago: University of Chicago Press.

Hart, S., Kropp, P., & Hare, R. (1988). Performance of psychopaths following conditional release from prison. *Journal of Consulting and Clinical Psychology, 56,* 227–232.

Heilbrun, K. (1997). Prediction versus management models relevant to risk assessment: The importance of legal decision-making context. *Law and Human Behavior, 21,* 347–359.

Heilbrun, K., Hart, S., Hare, R., Gustafson, D., Nunez, C., & White, A. (1998). Inpatient and postdischarge aggression in mentally disordered offenders: The role of psychopathy. *Journal of Interpersonal Violence, 13,* 514–527.

Heilbrun, K., & Peters, L. (2000). The efficacy and effectiveness of community treatment programmes in preventing crime and violence among those with severe mental illness in the community. In S. Hodgins (Ed.), *Effective prevention of crime and violence among the mentally ill.* Dordrecht, the Netherlands: Kluwer Academic.

Hemphill, J., & Hare, R. (1999). Psychopathy checklist factor scores and recidivism. *Issues in Criminological and Legal Psychology, 24,* 68–73.

Hemphill, J., Templeman, R., Wong, S., & Hare, R. (1998). Psychopathy and crime: Recidivism and criminal careers. In D. Cooke, A. Forth, & R. Hare, (Eds.), *Psychopathy: Theory, research, and implications for society* (pp. 374–399). Dordrecht, the Netherlands: Kluwer Academic.

Hiday, V. (1995). The social context of mental illness and violence. *Journal of Health and Social Behavior, 36,* 122–137.

Hill, C., Rogers, R., & Bickford, M. (1996). Predicting aggressive and socially disruptive behavior in a maximum security forensic psychiatric hospital. *Journal of Forensic Sciences, 51,* 56–59.

Hodgins, S. (1992). Mental disorder, intellectual deficiency and crime: Evidence from a birth cohort. *Archives of General Psychiatry, 49,* 476–483.

Hollingshead, A. & Redlich, F. (1958). *Social class and mental illness.* New York: Guilford Press.

Hoyer, G. (2000). Social services necessary for community treatment programmes designed to prevent crime and violence among persons with major mental disorders. In S. Hodgins (Ed.), *Effective prevention of crime and violence among the mentally ill.* Dordrecht, the Netherlands: Kluwer Academic Publishers.

Humphreys, M., Johnstone, E. MacMillan, J., & Taylor, P. (1992). Dangerous behaviour preceding first admissions for schizophrenia. *British Journal of Psychiatry, 161,* 501–505.

Janca, A., & Helzer, J. (1990). DSM-III-R criteria checklist. *DIS Newsletter, 7,* 17.

Junginger, J., Parks-Levy, J., & McGuire, L. (1998). Delusions and symptom-consistent violence. *Psychiatric Services, 49*, 218–220.

Kenrick, D., & Sheets, V. (1993). Homicidal fantasies. *Ethology and Sociology, 14*, 231–246.

Klassen, D., & O'Connor, W. (1988a). A prospective study of predictors of violence in adult male mental patients. *Law and Human Behavior, 12*, 143–158.

Klassen, D., & O'Connor, W. (1988b). Crime, inpatient admissions, and violence among male mental patients. *International Journal of Law and Psychiatry, 11*, 305–312.

Klassen, D., & O'Connor, W. (1990). Assessing the risk of violence in released mental patients: A cross-validation study. *Psychological Assessment: A Journal of Consulting and Clinical Psychology, 1*, 75–81.

Klassen, D., & O'Connor, W. (1994). Demographic and case history variables in risk assessment. In J. Monahan and H. Steadman (Eds.), *Violence and mental disorder: Developments in risk assessment* (pp. 229–257). Chicago: University of Chicago Press.

Konecni, V. (1975a). Annoyance, type and duration of post-annoyance activity, and aggression: The "cathartic effect." *Journal of Experimental Psychology: General, 104*, 76–102.

Konecni, V. (1975b). The mediation of aggressive behavior: Arousal level versus anger and cognitive labeling. *Journal of Personality and Social Psychology, 32*, 706–712.

Kozol, H., Boucher, R., & Garofalo, R. (1972). The diagnosis and treatment of dangerousness. *Crime and Delinquency, 18*, 371–392.

Kraemer, H., Kazdin, A., Offord, D., Kessler, R., Jensen, P., & Kupfer, D. (1997). Coming to terms with the terms of risk. *Archives of General Psychiatry, 54*, 337.

Land, K. C., McCall, P. L., & Cohen, L. E. (1990). Structural covariates of homicide rates: Are there any invariances across time and social space? *American Journal of Sociology, 95*, 922–963.

Land, K., & Nagin, D. (1996). Micro-models of criminal careers: A synthesis of the criminal careers and life course approaches via semiparametric mixed Poisson regression models, with empirical applications. *Journal of Quantitative Criminology, 12*, 163–191.

Lidz, C., Hoge, S., Gardner, W., Bennett, N., Monahan, J., Mulvey, E., & Roth, L. (1995). Perceived coercion in mental hospital admission: Pressures and process. *Archives of General Psychiatry, 52*:1034–1039.

Lidz, C., Mulvey, E., Apperson, L., Evanczuk, K., & Shea, S. (1992). Sources of disagreement among clinicians' assessments of dangerousness in a psychiatric emergency room. *International Journal of Law and Psychiatry, 15,* 237–250

Lidz, C., Mulvey, E., & Gardner, W. (1993). The accuracy of predictions of violence to others. *Journal of the American Medical Association, 269,* 1007–1011.

Lilienfeld, S. (1994). Conceptual problems in the assessment of psychopathy. *Clinical Psychology Review, 14,* 17–38.

Lilienfeld, S. (1998). Methodological advances and developments in the assessment of psychopathy. *Behaviour Research and Therapy, 36,* 99–125.

Link, B., Andrews, D., & Cullen, F. (1992). The violent and illegal behavior of mental patients reconsidered. *American Sociological Review, 57,* 275–292.

Link, B., Monahan, J., Stueve, A., & Cullen, F. (1999a). Real in their consequences: A sociological approach to understanding the association between psychotic symptoms and violence. *American Sociological Review, 64,* 316–332.

Link, B., Phelan, J., Bresnahan, M., Stueve, A., & Pescosolido, B. (1999b). Public conceptions of mental illness: Labels, causes, dangerousness, and social distance. *American Journal of Public Health, 89,* 1328–1333.

Link, B., & Stueve, A. (1994). Psychotic symptoms and the violent/illegal behavior of mental patients compared to community controls. In J. Monahan, & H. Steadman, (Eds.), *Violence and mental disorder: Developments in risk assessment* (pp. 137–159). Chicago: University of Chicago Press.

Lösel, F. (1998). Treatment and management of psychopaths. In D. Cooke, A. Forth, & R. Hare (Eds.), *Psychopathy: Theory, research, and implications for society* (pp. 303–354). Dordrecht, the Netherlands: Kluwer Academic.

Lynam, D. (1996). Early identification of chronic offenders: Who is the fledgling psychopath? *Psychological Bulletin, 120,* 209–234.

MacDonald, J. (1967). Homicidal threats. *American Journal of Psychiatry, 124,* 475.

Malamuth, N. (1998). The confluence model as an organizing framework for research on sexually aggressive men: Risk moderators, imagined aggression, and pornography consumption. In R. Geen, & E. Donnerstein, (Eds.), *Human aggression: Theories, research, and implications for social policy* (pp. 229–245). New York: Academic Press.

Martell, D., & Dietz, P. (1992). Mentally disordered offenders who push or attempt to push victims onto subway tracks in New York City. *Archives of General Psychiatry, 49,* 472–475.

McNiel, D. (1994). Hallucinations and violence. In J. Monahan, & H. Steadman, (Eds.), *Violence and mental disorder: Developments in risk assessment* (pp. 83–202). Chicago: University of Chicago Press.

McNiel, D. (1998). Empirically based clinical evaluation and management of the potentially violent patient. In P. Kleespies, (Ed.), *Emergencies in mental health practice: Evaluation and management* (pp. 95–116). New York: Guilford Press.

McNiel, D., & Binder, R. (1994). Screening for risk of inpatient violence: Validation of an actuarial tool. *Law and Human Behavior, 18,* 579–586.

McNiel, D., & Binder, R. (1995). Correlates of accuracy in the assessment of psychiatric inpatients' risk of violence. *American Journal of Psychiatry, 148,* 1317–1321.

McNiel, D., Eisner, J., and Binder, R. (2000). The relationship between command hallucinations and violence. *Psychiatric Services, 51,* 1288–1292.

McNiel, D., Lam, J., & Binder, R. (in press). Relevance of inter-rater agreement to violence risk assessment. *Journal of Consulting and Clinical Psychology.*

McNiel, D., Sandberg, D., & Binder, R. (1998). The relationship between confidence and accuracy in clinical assessment of psychiatric patients' potential for violence. *Law and Human Behavior, 22,* 655–669.

Meehl, P. (1954). *Clinical versus statistical prediction: A theoretical analysis and a review of the evidence.* Minneapolis: University of Minnesota.

Melton, G., Petrila, J., Poythress, N., & Slobogin, C. (1997). *Psychological evaluations for the courts: A handbook for mental health professionals and lawyers* (2nd ed.). New York: Guilford Press.

Menzies, R., & Webster, C. (1995). Construction and validation of risk-assessments in a six-year follow-up of forensic patients: A tridimensional analysis. *Journal of Consulting and Clinical Psychology, 63,* 766–778.

Menzies, R., Webster, C., & Sepejak, D. (1985). The dimensions of dangerousness: Evaluating the accuracy of psychometric predictions of violence among forensic patients. *Law and Human Behavior, 9,* 49–70.

Miethe, T. D., & McDowall, D. (1993). Contextual effects in models of criminal victimization. *Social Forces, 71,* 741–759.

Monahan, J. (1981). *The clinical prediction of violent behavior.* Washington, DC: Government Printing Office.

Monahan, J. (1993). Limiting therapist exposure to *Tarasoff* liability: Guidelines for risk containment. *American Psychologist, 48,* 242–250.

Monahan, J. (2000a). Violence risk assessment: Scientific validity and evidentiary admissibility. *Washington and Lee Law Review, 57,* 901–918.

Monahan, J. (2000b). Clinical and actuarial predictions of violence. In D. Faigman, D. Kaye, M. Saks, & J. Sanders, (Eds.), *Modern scientific evidence: The law and science of expert testimony* (pp. 300–318). St. Paul, MN: West.

Monahan, J., & Appelbaum, P. (2000). Reducing violence risk: Diagnostically based clues from the MacArthur Violence Risk Assessment Study. In S. Hodgins (Ed.),

Effective prevention of crime and violence among the mentally ill (pp. 19–34). Dordrecht, the Netherlands: Kluwer Academic.

Monahan, J., Appelbaum, P., Mulvey, E., Robbins, P., & Lidz, C. (1994). Ethical and legal duties in conducting research on violence: Lessons from the MacArthur Risk Assessment Study. *Violence and Victims 8,* 380–390.

Monahan, J., & Steadman, H. (Eds.). (1994). *Violence and mental disorder: Developments in risk assessment.* Chicago: University of Chicago Press.

Monahan, J., & Steadman, H. (1996). Violent storms and violent people: How meteorology can inform risk communication in mental health law. *American Psychologist, 51,* 931–938.

Monahan, J., Steadman, H., Appelbaum, P., Robbins, P., Mulvey, E., Silver, E., Roth, L., and Grisso, T. (2000). Developing a clinically useful actuarial tool for assessing violence risk. *British Journal of Psychiatry, 176,* 312–319.

Mooney, C., & Duval, R. (1993). *Bootstrapping: A nonparametric approach to statistical inference.* Newbury Park, CA: Sage.

Mossman, D. (1994). Assessing predictions of violence: Being accurate about accuracy. *Journal of Consulting and Clinical Psychology, 62,* 783–792.

Mossman, D. (2000). Commentary: Assessing the risk of violence—Are "accurate" predictions useful? *Journal of the American Academy of Psychiatry and the Law, 28,* 272–281.

Mullen, P. (1997). Assessing risk of interpersonal violence in the mentally ill. *Advances in Psychiatric Treatment, 3,* 166–173.

Mullen, P. (2000). Forensic mental health. *British Journal of Psychiatry, 176,* 307–311.

Mulvey, E., Blumstein, A., & Cohen, J. (1986). Reframing the research question of mental patient criminality. *International Journal of Law and Psychiatry, 9,* 57–65.

Mulvey, E., & Lidz, C. (1985). Back to basics: A critical analysis of dangerousness research in a new legal environment. *Law and Human Behavior, 9,* 209–218.

Mulvey, E., & Lidz, C. (1993). Measuring patient violence in dangerousness research. *Law and Human Behavior, 17,* 277–288.

Mulvey, E., Shaw, E., & Lidz, C. (1994). Why use multiple sources in research on patient violence in the community? *Criminal Behaviour and Mental Health, 4,* 253–258.

Nagin, D., & Land, K. (1993). Age, criminal careers, and population heterogeneity: Specification and estimation of a nonparametric, mixed Poisson model. *Criminology, 31,* 327–359.

Nagin, D., & Tremblay, R. (1999). Trajectories of boys' physical aggression, opposition, and hyperactivity on the path to physical violence and nonviolent juvenile delinquency. *Child Development, 70,* 1181–1196.

Nelson, L. (1977). Tables for testing ordered alternatives in an analysis of variance. *Biometrika, 64,* 333–336.

Newhill, C., Mulvey, E., & Lidz, C. (1995). Characteristics of violence in the community by female patients seen in a psychiatric emergency service. *Psychiatric Services 46,* 785–795.

Nolan, K., Volavka, J., Mohr, P., & Czobor, P. (1999). Psychopathy and violent behavior among patients with schizophrenia or schizoaffective disorder. *Psychiatric Services, 50,* 787–792.

Novaco, R. (1994). Anger as a risk factor for violence among the mentally disordered. In J. Monahan, & H. Steadman, (Eds.), *Violence and mental disorder: Developments in risk assessment* (pp. 21–59). Chicago: University of Chicago Press.

Novaco, R. (1997). Remediating anger and aggression with violent offenders. *Legal and Criminological Psychology, 2,* 77–88.

Ohlin, L. (1951). *Selection for parole.* New York: Russell Sage.

Otto, R., Poythress, N., Nicholson, R., Edens, J., Monahan, J., Bonnie, R., Hoge, S., & Eisenberg, M. (1998). Psychometric properties of the MacArthur Competence Assessment Tool—Criminal Adjudication. *Psychological Assessment, 10,* 435–443.

Overall, J. (1988). The Brief Psychiatric Rating Scale (BPRS): Recent developments in ascertainment and scaling. *Psychopharmacology Bulletin, 24,* 97–99.

Overall, J., & Gorham, D. (1962). The Brief Psychiatric Rating Scale. *Psychological Reports, 10,* 799–812.

Patrick, C., Bradley, M., & Lang, P. (1993). Emotion in the criminal psychopath: Startle reflex modulation. *Journal of Abnormal Psychology, 102,* 82–92.

Pescosolido, B., Monahan, J., Link, B., Stueve, A., & Kikuzawa, S. (1999). The public's view of the competence, dangerousness and need for legal coercion among persons with mental illness. *American Journal of Public Health, 89,* 1339–1345.

Pfohl, B., Blum, N., Zimmerman, M., & Stangl, D. (1989). *The Structured Interview for DSM-III Personality: SIDP-R.* Iowa City: University of Iowa.

Phelan, J., Link, B., Stueve, A., & Pescosolido, B. (2000). Public conceptions of mental illness in 1950 and 1996: What is mental illness and is it to be feared? *Journal of Health and Social Behavior, 41,* 188–207.

Pilkonis, P., & Klein, K. (1997). Commentary on the assessment and diagnosis of antisocial behavior and personality. In D. Stoff, J. Breiling, J. & Maser, (Eds.), *Handbook of antisocial behavior* (pp. 109–112). New York: John Wiley & Sons.

Quinsey, V., Harris, G., Rice, M., & Cormier, C. (1998). *Violent offenders: Appraising and managing risk.* Washington, DC: American Psychological Association.

Quinsey, V., & Maguire, A. (1986). Maximum security psychiatric patients: Actuarial and clinical prediction of dangerousness. *Journal of Interpersonal Violence, 1,* 143–171.

Quinsey, V., Warneford, A., Pruesse, M., & Link, N. (1975). Released Oak Ridge patients: A follow-up study of review board discharges. *British Journal of Criminology, 15,* 264–270.

Reiss, A., & Roth, J. (1993). *Understanding and preventing violence.* Washington, DC: National Academy Press.

Rice, M., & Harris, G. (1995a). Psychopathy, schizophrenia, alcohol abuse, and violent recidivism. *International Journal of Law and Psychiatry, 18,* 333–342.

Rice, M., & Harris, G. (1995b). Violent recidivism: Assessing predictive validity. *Journal of Consulting and Clinical Psychology, 63,* 737–748.

Rice, M., & Harris, G. (1997). The treatment of mentally disordered offenders. *Psychology, Public Policy, and Law, 3,* 126–183.

Rice, M., Harris, G., & Quinsey, V. (1990). A follow-up of rapists assessed in a maximum security psychiatric facility. *Journal of Interpersonal Violence, 4,* 435–448.

Robins, L. (1966). *Deviant children grown up.* Baltimore, MD: Williams & Williams.

Robins, L., Helzer, J., Croughan, J., Williams, J., & Spitzer, R. (Eds.). (1981). *National Institute of Mental Health Diagnostic Interview Schedule* (version 3). Washington, DC: Government Printing Office.

Robbins, P., Monahan, J., & Silver, E. (2000). Mental disorder, violence, and gender. (Submitted for publication.)

Rogers, R. (1995). *Diagnostic and structured interviewing: A handbook for psychologists.* Odessa, FL: Psychological Assessment Resources.

Rose, S., Peabody, C., & Stratigeas, B. (1991). Undetected abuse among intensive case management clients. *Hospital & Community Psychiatry, 42,* 499–503.

Rosenfeld, E., Huesmann, L., Eron, L., & Torney-Purta, J. (1982). Measuring fantasy behavior in children. *Journal of Personality and Social Psychology, 42,* 347–366.

Roth, L. (1979). A commitment law for patients, doctors, and lawyers. *American Journal of Psychiatry, 136,* 1121–1127.

Roth, L. (1985). *Clinical treatment of the violent person.* Washington, DC: Government Printing Office.

Rubin, D. B. (1997). *Nonrandomized comparative clinical studies, Proceedings of the International Conference on Nonrandomized Comparative Clinical Studies.* Heidelberg, April 10–11.

Rudnick, A. (1999). Relation between command hallucinations and dangerous behavior. *Journal of the American Academy of Psychiatry and the Law, 27,* 253–257.

Salekin, R., Rogers, R., & Sewell, K. (1996). A review and meta-analysis of the Psychopathy Checklist and Psychopathy Checklist–Revised: Predictive validity of dangerousness. *Clinical Psychology: Science and Practice, 3,* 203–215.

Sampson, R. J., & Lauritsen, J. L. (1994). Violent victimization and offending: Individual-, situational-, and community-level risk factors. In A. J. Reiss, & J. A. Roth (Eds.), *Understanding and preventing violence* (Vol. 3, pp. 1–114). Washington, DC: National Academy Press.

Sampson, R. J., Raudenbush, S. W., & Earls, F. (1997). Neighborhoods and violent crime: A multilevel study of collective efficacy. *Science, 277,* 918–924.

Segal, S., Watson, M., Goldfinger, S., & Averbuck, D. (1988a). Civil commitment in the psychiatric emergency room I: The assessment of dangerousness by emergency room clinicians. *Archives of General Psychiatry, 45,* 748–752.

Segal, S., Watson, M., Goldfinger, S., & Averbuck, D. (1988b). Civil commitment in the psychiatric emergency room II: Mental disorder indicators and three dangerousness criteria. *Archives of General Psychiatry, 45,* 753–758.

Sepejak, D., Menzies, R., Webster, C., & Jensen, F. (1983). Clinical predictions of dangerousness: Two-year follow-up of 408 pre-trial forensic cases. *Bulletin of the American Academy of Psychiatry and the Law, 11,* 171–181.

Serin, R., & Amos, N. (1995). The role of psychopathy in the assessment of dangerousness. *International Journal of Law and Psychiatry, 18,* 231–238.

Shah, S. (1978). Dangerousness and mental illness: Some conceptual, prediction, and policy dilemmas. In Frederick, C. (Ed.), *Dangerous behavior: A problem in law and mental health* (pp. 153–191). Washington, DC: Government Printing Office.

Silver, E. (1995). Punishment or treatment?: Comparing the lengths of confinement of successful and unsuccessful insanity defendants. *Law and Human Behavior, 19,* 375–388.

Silver, E. (2000). Race, neighborhood disadvantage, and violence among persons with mental disorders: The importance of contextual measurement. *Law and Human Behavior, 24,* 449–456.

Silver, E. (2000). Extending social disorganization theory: A multilevel approach to the study of violence among persons with mental illnesses. *Criminology, 38,* 301–332.

Silver, E., Mulvey, E. P., & Monahan, J. (1999). Assessing violence risk among discharged psychiatric patients: Toward an ecological approach. *Law and Human Behavior, 23,* 235–253.

Silver, E., Smith, W. R., & Banks, S. (2000). Constructing actuarial devices for predicting recidivism: A comparison of methods. *Criminal Justice and Behavior, 27*, 732–763.

Silver, J., & Caton, C. (1989). *Head injury questionnaire.* Unpublished manuscript, Columbia University.

Silver, R. (1996). Sex differences in the solitary assaultive fantasies of delinquent and nondelinquent adolescents. *Adolescence, 31*, 543–552.

Skeem, J., & Mulvey, E. (in press-a). Psychopathy and community violence among civil psychiatric patients: Results from the MacArthur Violence Risk Assessment Study. *Journal of Consulting and Clinical Psychology.*

Skeem, J., & Mulvey, E. (in press-b). Assessing the violence potential of mentally disordered offenders being treated in the community. In A. Buchanan, (Ed.), *Care of the mentally disordered offender in the community.* Oxford: Oxford University Press.

Slovic, P., Monahan, J., & MacGregor, D. (2000). Violence risk assessment and risk communication: The effects of using actual cases, providing instruction, and employing probability versus frequency formats. *Law and Human Behavior, 24*, 271–296.

SPSS, Inc. (1993). SPSS for Windows CHAID (Release 6.0) [Computer software]. Chicago: SPSS.

Steadman, H. (1977). A new look at recidivism among Patuxent inmates. *The Bulletin on the American Academy of Psychiatry and the Law, 5*, 200–209.

Steadman, H., & Cocozza, J. (1974). *Careers of the criminally insane.* Lexington, MA: Lexington Books.

Steadman, H., Monahan, J., Appelbaum, P., Grisso, T., Mulvey, E., Roth, L., Robbins, P., & Klassen, D. (1994). Designing a new generation of risk assessment research. In Monahan, J., & Steadman, H. (Eds.), *Violence and mental disorder: Developments in risk assessment* (pp. 297–318). Chicago: University of Chicago Press.

Steadman, H., McGreevy, M., Morrissey, J., Callahan, L., Robbins, P. & Cirincione, C. (1993). *Before and after Hinckley: Evaluating insanity defense reform.* New York: Guilford.

Steadman, H., & Morrissey, J. (1982). Predicting violent behavior: A note on a cross-validation study. *Social Forces, 61*, 475–483.

Steadman, H., Mulvey, E., Monahan, J., Robbins, P., Appelbaum, P., Grisso, T., Roth, L., & Silver, E. (1998). Violence by people discharged from acute psychiatric inpatient facilities and by others in the same neighborhoods. *Archives of General Psychiatry, 55*, 393–401.

Steadman, H., & Silver, E. (2000). Immediate precursors to violence among persons with mental illness. A return to a situational perspective. In S. Hodgins (Ed.), *Effective prevention of crime and violence among the mentally ill* (pp. 35–48). Dordrecht, the Netherlands: Kluwer Academic.

Steadman, H., Silver, E., Monahan, J., Appelbaum, P., Robbins, P., Mulvey, E., Grisso, T., Roth, L., & Banks, S. (2000). A classification tree approach to the development of actuarial violence risk assessment tools. *Law and Human Behavior, 24(1)*, 83–100.

Steffensmeier, D., & Allen, E. (1996). Gender and crime: Toward a gendered theory of criminal offending. *Annual Review of Sociology, 22*, 459–487.

Steinberg, D., & Colla, P. (1995). CART: *Tree-structured non-parametric data analysis*. San Diego: Salford Systems, 1995.

Steury, E. H., and Choinski, M. (1995). "Normal" crimes and mental disorder: A two-group comparison of deadly and dangerous felonies. *International Journal of Law and Psychiatry, 18* (2), 183–207.

Stone, A. (1975). *Mental health and the law: A system in transition*. Washington, DC: Government Printing Office.

Strand, S., Belfrage, H., Fransson, G., & Levander, S. (1999). Clinical and risk management factors in risk prediction of mentally disordered offenders — more important than historical data? *Legal and Criminological Psychology, 4*, 67–76.

Surgeon General (1999). *Mental health: a report of the Surgeon General*. Washington, DC: Office of the Surgeon General.

Swanson, J., Borum, R., Swartz, M., & Hiday, V. (1999). Violent behavior preceding hospitalization among persons with severe mental illness. *Law and Human Behavior, 23*, 185–204.

Swanson, J., Borum, R., Swartz, M., & Monahan, J. (1996). Psychotic symptoms and disorders and the risk of violent behavior in the community. *Criminal Behaviour and Mental Health, 6*, 317–338.

Swanson, J., Estroff, S., Swartz, M., Borum, R., Lachicotte, W., Zimmer, C., & Wagner, R. (1997). Violence and severe mental disorder in clinical and community populations: The effects of psychotic symptoms, comorbidity, and lack of treatment. *Psychiatry, 60*, 1–22.

Swanson, J., Holzer, C., Ganju, V., & Jono, R. (1990). Violence and psychiatric disorder in the community: Evidence from the epidemiological catchment area surveys. *Hospital and Community Psychiatry, 41*, 761–770.

Swanson, J., Swartz, M., Borum, R., Hiday, V., Wagner, R., & Burns, B. (2000). Involuntary out-patient commitment and reduction of violent behaviour in persons with severe mental illness. *British Journal of Psychiatry, 176*, 324–331.

Swartz, M., Swanson, J., Hiday, V., Borum, R., Wagner, H., & Burns, B. (1998).

Violence and severe mental illness: The effects of substance abuse and non-adherence to medication. *American Journal of Psychiatry, 155,* 226–231.

Swartz, M., Swanson, J., Wagner, H., Burns, B., Hiday, V., & Borum, R. (1999). Can involuntary outpatient commitment reduce hospital recidivism? Findings from a randomized trail with severly mentally ill individuals. *American Journal of Psychiatry, 156,* 1968–1975.

Swets, J. (1988) Measuring the accuracy of diagnostic systems. *Science, 240,* 1285–1293.

Swets, J., Dawes, R., and Monahan, J. (2000). Psychological science can improve diagnostic decisions. *Psychological Science in the Public Interest, 1,* 1–26.

Tabachnick, B., & Fidell, L. (1996). *Using multivariate statistics* (3rd ed.). New York: Harper Collins.

Tardiff, K., Marzuk, P. M., Leon, A. C., & Portera, L. (1997). A prospective study of violence by psychiatric patients after hospital discharge. *Psychiatric Services, 48,* 678–681.

Taylor, P. (1985). Motives for offending among violent and psychotic men. *British Journal of Psychiatry, 147,* 491–498.

Taylor, P. (1993). Schizophrenia and crime: Distinctive patterns in association. In S. Hodgins (Ed.), *Mental disorder and crime* (pp. 63–85). Newbury Park, CA: Sage.

Taylor, P. (1998). When symptoms of psychosis drive serious violence. *Social Psychiatry and Psychiatric Epidemiology, 33,* 47–54.

Taylor, P., Garety, P., Buchanan, A., Reed, A., Wessely, A., Ray, K., Dunn, G., & Grubin, D. (1994). Delusions and violence. In Monahan, J., & Steadman, H. (Eds.), *Violence and mental disorder: Developments in risk assessment.* Chicago: University of Chicago Press.

Thornberry, T., & Jacoby, J. (1979). *The criminally insane: A community follow-up of mentally ill offenders.* Chicago: University of Chicago Press.

Tiihonen, J., Isohanni, M., Rasanen, P., Koiranen, M., & Moring, J. (1997). Specific major mental disorders and criminality: A 26-year prospective study of the 1966 northern Finland birth cohort. *American Journal of Psychiatry, 154,* 840–845.

Toch, H. (1998). Psychopathy or antisocial personality in forensic settings. In T. Millon, E. Simonsen, M. Birket-Smith, & R. Davis (Eds.), *Psychopathy: Antisocial, criminal, and violent behavior* (pp. 144–158). New York: Guilford Press.

Toch, H., & Adams, K. (1994). *The disturbed violent offender (Rev. ed.).* Washington, DC: American Psychological Association.

Virkkunen, M. (1974). Observations on violence in schizophrenia. *Acta Psychiatrica Scandinavica, 50,* 145–151.

Wallace, C., Mullen, P., Burgess, P., Palmer, S., Ruschena, & Brown, C. (1998).

Serious criminal offending and mental disorder: Case linkage study. *British Journal of Psychiatry*, *172*, 477–484.

Webster, C., Douglas, K., Belfrage, & Link, B. (2000). Capturing change. An approach to managing violence and improving mental health. In S. Hodgins (Ed.), *Effective prevention of crime and violence among the mentally ill* (pp. 119–144). Dordrecht, the Netherlands: Kluwer Academic.

Webster, C., Douglas, K., Eaves, D., & Hart, S. (1995). *HCR-20: Assessing risk for violence* (version 2). Vancouver: Simon Fraser University.

Webster, C., Harris, G., Rice, M., Cormier, C, & Quinsey, V. (1994). *The violence prediction scheme: Assessing dangerousness in high risk men*. Toronto: Centre of Criminology, University of Toronto.

Wessely, S. (1997). The epidemiology of crime, violence and schizophrenia. *British Journal of Psychiatry*, *170*, 8–11.

Wessely, S., & Taylor, P. (1991). Madness and crime: Criminology versus psychiatry. *Criminal Behaviour and Mental Health*, *1*, 193–228.

White, H. (1997). Alcohol, illicit drugs, and violence. In D. Stoff, J. Breiling, & J. Maser (Eds.), *Handbook of antisocial behavior* (pp. 511–523). New York: John Wiley & Sons.

Widiger, T., Cadoret, R., Hare, R., Robins, L., Rutherford, M., Zanarini, M., Alterman, A., Apple, M., Corbitt, E., Forth, A., Hart, S., Kultermann, J., Woody, G., & Frances, A. (1996). DSM-IV antisocial personality disorder field trial. *Journal of Abnormal Psychology*, *105*, 3–16.

Widom, C. (1989a). Does violence beget violence? A critical examination of the literature. *Psychological Bulletin*, *106*, 3–28.

Widom, C. (1989b). The cycle of violence. *Science*, *244*, 160–166.

Wilson, J., & Herrnstein, R. (1985). *Crime and human nature*. New York: Simon & Schuster.

Yesavage, J. A. (1984). Correlates of dangerous behavior by schizophrenics in hospitals. *Journal of Psychiatric Research*, *18*, 225–233.

Yesavage, J., Becker, J., Werner, P., Patton, M., Seeman, K., Brunsting, D., & Mills, M. (1983). Family conflict, psychopathology, and dangerous behavior by schizophrenic inpatients. *Psychiatry Research*, *8*, 271–280.

INDEX